Aesthetic Microcannula
for Cosmetic Injectable Fillers

by Garry R. Lee, MD

Aesthetic Microcannula for Cosmetic Injectable Fillers
by Garry R. Lee, MD
Medical Director of Look Younger MD
2610 W. Horizon Ridge Pkwy. #100
Las Vegas, NV 89052
United States of America
(702) 938-0190

www.LookYoungerMD.com
Email: LookYoungerMD@gmail.com

Book Layout and Design
by Linda A. Bell
HeartToHeartStudio.com

Medical / Education & Training: advanced anti-bruising cosmetic injection techniques/ Garry R. Lee, MD

ISBN-13: 978-0-578-52874-8

Printed in the United States of America

Disclaimer

The content presented is for informational purposes only, is a compilation of the personal clinical experiences of the author, and is not definitive in nature or necessarily representative of any of the organizations for which Dr. Lee is an instructor. Off-label uses of FDA Approved products and devices are described and stringent application of current FDA guidelines should be observed. Readers should verify all information and complete hands-on preceptor training by highly proficient clinicians before application of any of the procedures described herein to patients. Consequently we disclaim any liability of any kind in any circumstance for any direct or indirect economic loss or damage for any revenue or loss of profit – and that we do not make any express, implied, or statutory representations, guarantees, warranties, conditions and obligations.

Acknowledgements

I wish to express my profound thanks to my patients who have volunteered to model our latest concepts knowing full well that they were the first to have ever done so, and from whom we have learned as much from what does not work – as what does. I also wish to thank the editors of our magazine publications who have given permission for me to use material from the issues of my published articles: *PRiME: the International Journal of Aesthetic & Anti-Aging Medicine, MedEsthetics, and The Aesthetic Guide.*

My appreciation also goes to those who have afforded me the signal privilege of teaching doctors and nurses on their behalf, including *Allergan, Galderma* (formerly *Medicis), Eclipse, the American Society of Cosmetic Physicians, The Aesthetic Show, The Canadian Academy of Aesthetic Medicine, Vegas Cosmetic Surgery & Aesthetic Dermatology, Aesthetic Everything, and The American Academy of Anti-Aging Medicine.* I also wish to thank AccuVein,™ PRO-NOX,™ Tom & Michael O'Brien, and Dr. Charles Runels of the Cellular Medicine Association for providing us with invaluable information.

My special appreciation is to Editor Linda Bell, TSK by *Air-Tite*, Carol Collins, MD, Mariale Foley, MD, Marcus Peterson, MD, FACS, and the dedicated and forbearing staff of Look Younger MD: Winona Sylvia, Jennifer Ivari, Judi Rush, and Jenna Shipman.

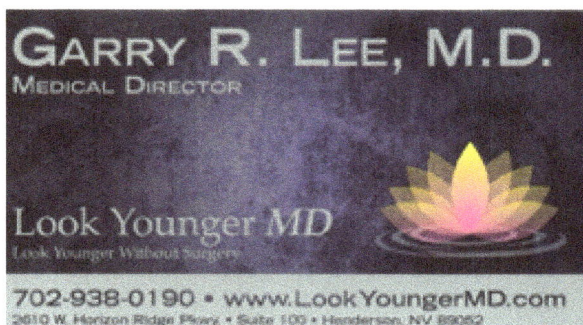

Look Younger MD

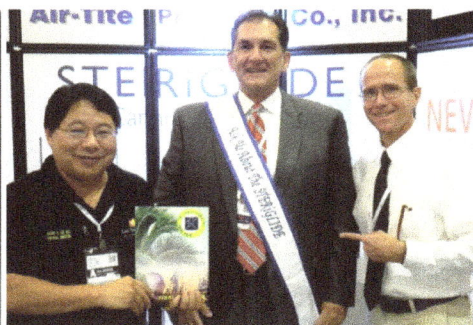

Air-Tite: Craig Johnson & Neil Granache

Disclosures: Garry R. Lee, MD, teaches physicians, nurses, and physician assistants, cosmetic procedures for Allergan, Galderma, TSK by Air-Tite, AccuVein,™ PRO-NOX,™ The Cellular Medicine Association, The American MedAesthetic Association, and Eclipse.

Contents

Contents

Dedication

To Super-Mom Ellen… and to Arwen, the Elf Warrior Princess.

Come as You Are
Leave as You Want to Be
Look Younger Without Surgery

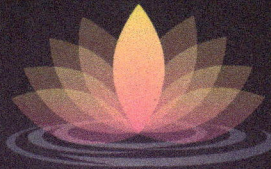

Preface

The way in which we use aesthetic microcannula for cosmetic filler injections has evolved so rapidly since the advent of *The First Book of Aesthetic MicroCannula for Cosmetic Fillers & Local Anesthesia (MILA)*[1] in 2016, that the 2nd Edition originally conceptualized has instead become our second book: *Aesthetic Microcannula for Cosmetic Injectable Fillers.* Indeed, the practical applications as well as the limitations of microcannula have become more evident leading to the elimination of old techniques for new, particularly since we have since refined our approach to one which more specifically targets the underlying anatomical changes of aging.

This book is for the physicians, nurses, and physician assistants who have dedicated their professional lives to achieving only the very best cosmetic injection practices on behalf of the patients who have honored us all with the privilege of their care.

The hypodermic needle has long dominated the parenteral delivery of modern medicine since 1853, when Scottish surgeon Alexander Wood devised a hollow metal needle on a syringe to inject medication into his patients.[2] Hence, it was only to be expected that when cosmetic wrinkle fillers were developed, that they would follow this conventional route.

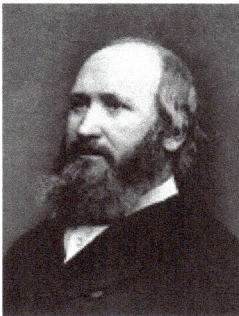

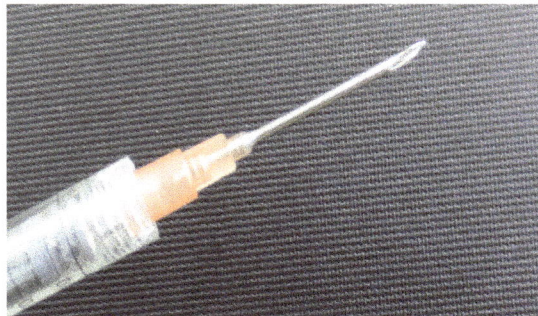

Dr. Alexander Wood (1817-1884) of Edinburgh; The Traditional Sharp Tip Hypodermic Needle

However, now that more cosmetic physicians, physician assistants, and nurses are transitioning from the exclusive use of the hypodermic needle to the predominate use of the aesthetic microcannula, it is time to update with our new book on current applications and techniques.

Our approach is to be as simple and as pictorial as possible, for the busy clinician who wants a quick reference to get the job done as expeditiously and as well as possible. Our focus has been my preferences among the most popular manufactured cosmetic injectable fillers which dominate the industry today instead of an overview of all approaches and all products. Excluded are products and techniques which I consider to be of excessive risk or which are deemed less effective or little used in 2019. Of increasing importance has been the use of hyaluronidase Off-Label for the accidental intravascular injection of hyaluronic acid filler as well as for aesthetic sculpting.

We have the honor to present in 2019, *Aesthetic Microcannula for Cosmetic Injectable Fillers.*

Injecting Cosmetic Fillers

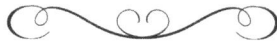

Introduction to Microcannula

The eternal quest has always been to look our very best…with the least expense, discomfort, risk, inconvenience, and healing time.

On one extreme, the realm of plastic surgery has refined to the point that what we can do today seems almost miraculous by previous standards. The skill of the surgeon has reached nearly inconceivable heights, though the latest advances will ultimately be in the unmatched precision of robotic surgery – with human guidance – supplemented with the evolving enhancement of artificial intelligence. Nevertheless, traditional plastic surgery today in conjunction with general anesthesia is generally the most expensive, most uncomfortable, and highest risk cosmetic procedure with the longest patient recovery time.

Concurrent with this progression has been the evolution of increasingly effective non-surgical aesthetic procedures such as neuromodulators (e.g. Botox Cosmetic® and Dysport®), lasers, intense pulsed light (IPL), radio-frequency (RF), microneedling, platelet-rich plasma (PRP) – as well as cosmetic injectable wrinkle fillers, threadlifts, and other energy devices

The use of non-permanent cosmetic injectable fillers to lift facial wrinkles has grown tremendously since the introduction of collagen, but especially since Medicis (now Galderma) introduced Restylane® in December of 2003, the first NASHA (non-animal-sourced hyaluronic acid gel) hyaluronic acid injectable product.[3]

Since then, a parade of other manufactured cosmetic fillers[4] have been introduced into the USA such as Juvederm,® Restylane Lyft® (formerly Perlane®), Radiesse,® Juvederm Voluma,® Juvederm Vobella,® Sculptra,® Restylane Refyne,® Restylane Defyne,® Revanesse® Versa,™ and Belotero Balance® – with each product attempting to outperform the others in duration of action, smoothness, elasticity with movement, ease of injection, and ability to stimulate the production of native collagen.

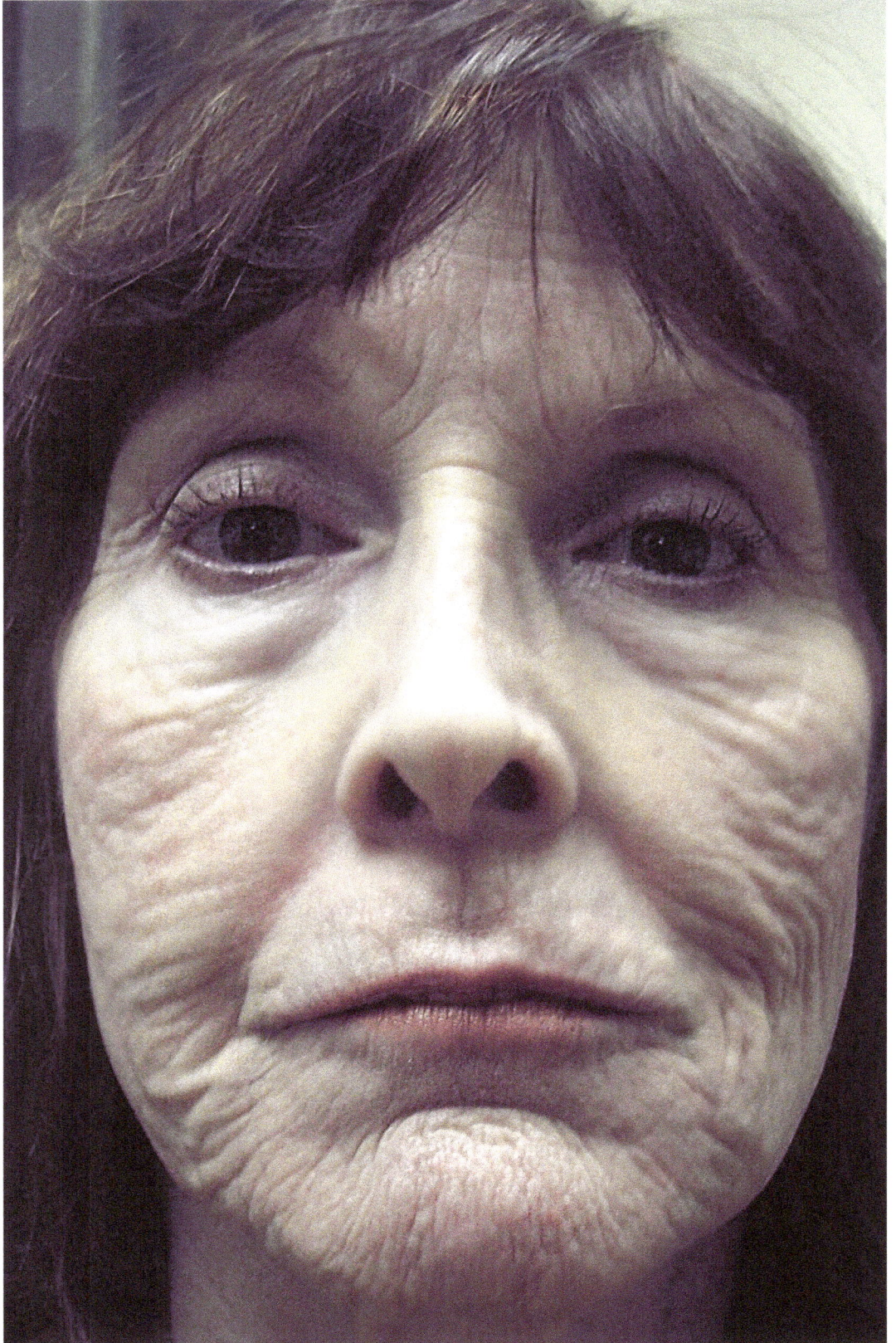

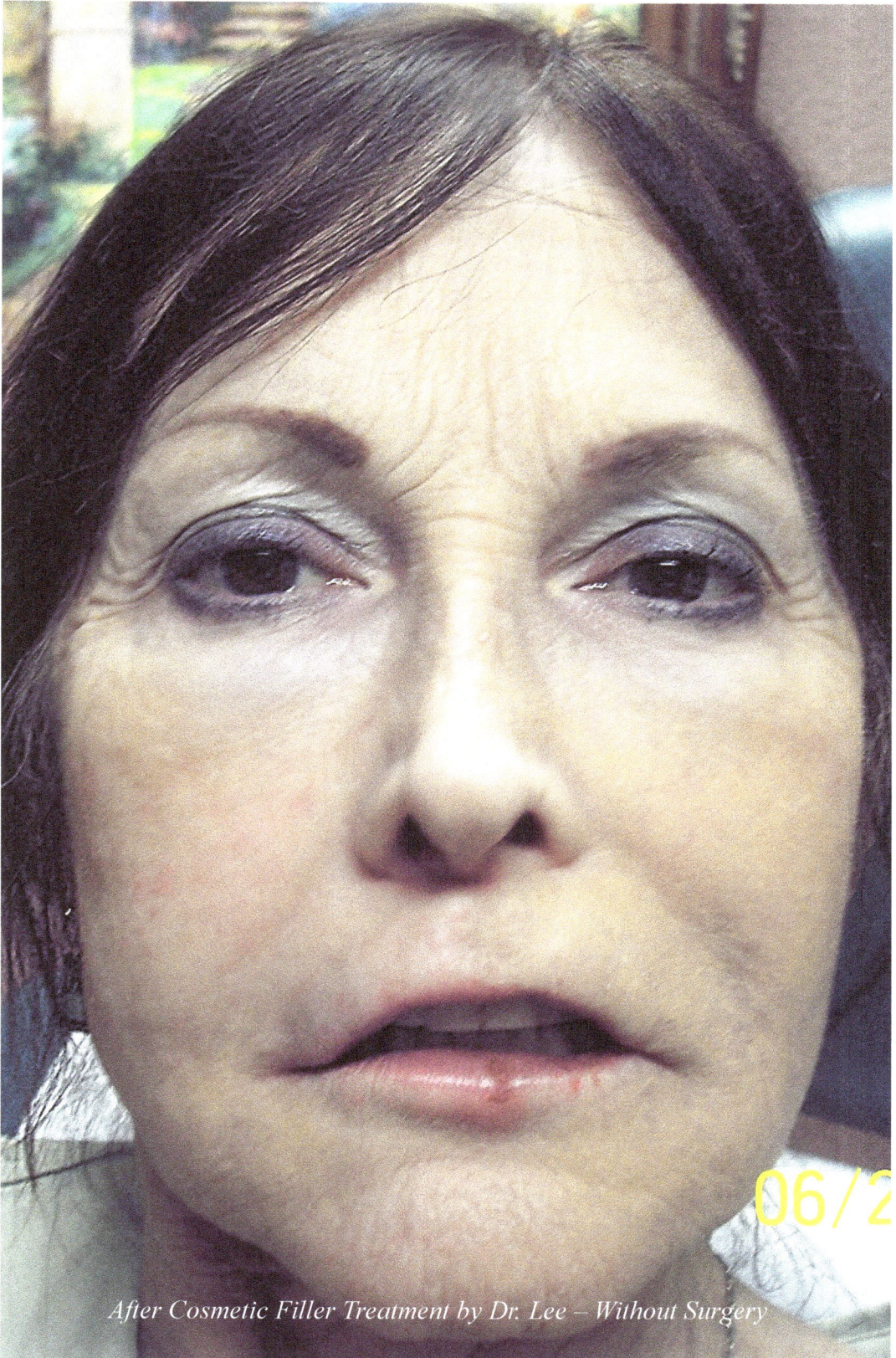

After Cosmetic Filler Treatment by Dr. Lee – Without Surgery

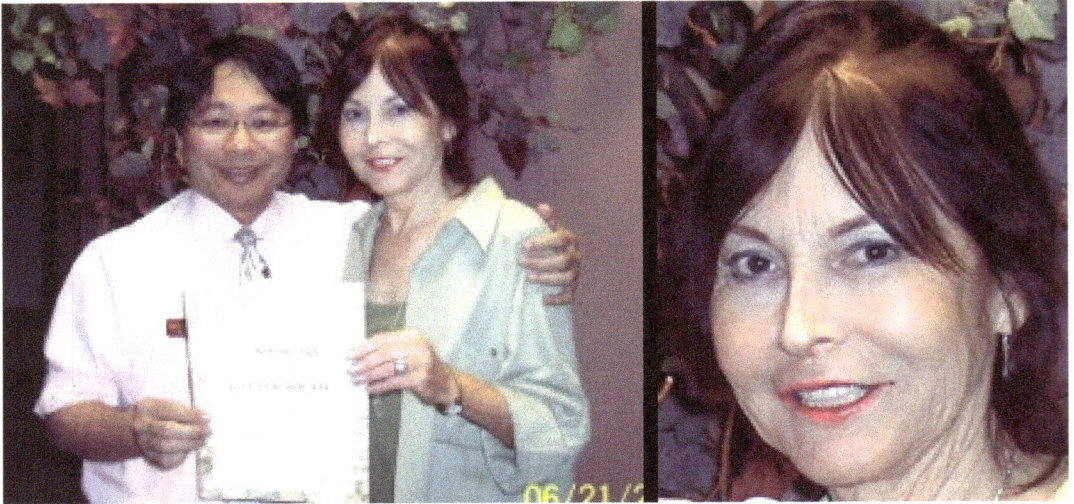

Traditionally, the use of hypodermic needles was the golden standard for cosmetic filler injections as technological innovations focused only upon improvements in the nature and duration of action of the fillers themselves.

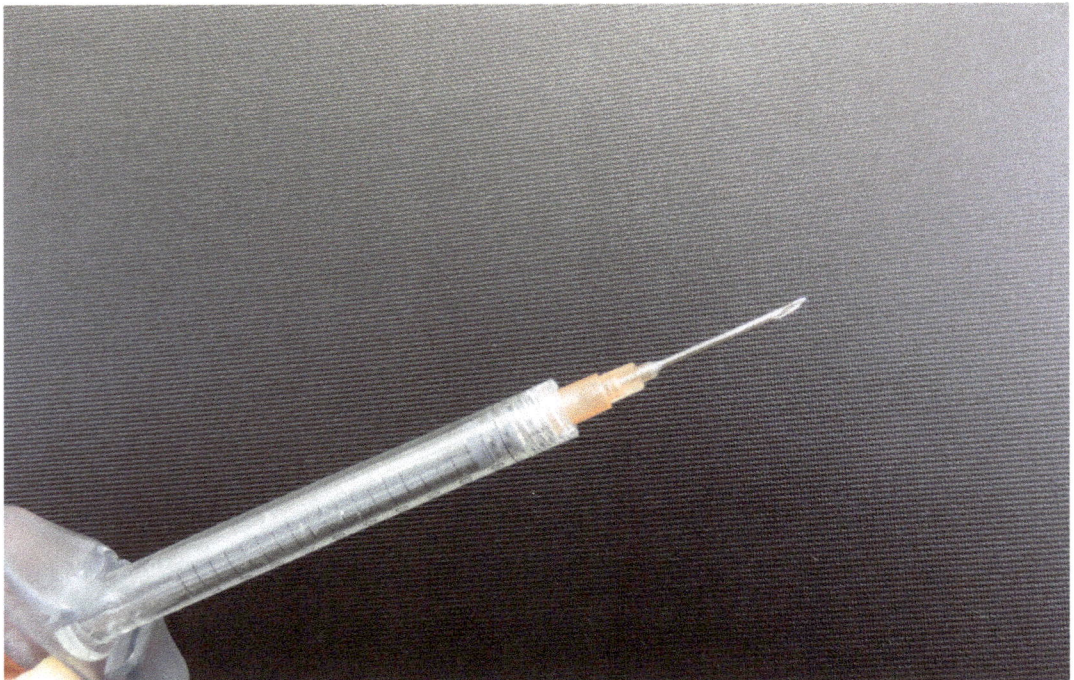

Unfortunately, bruising and swelling were more expected than not and it was not uncommon for patients to have as much apprehension for the sequelae as the treatment itself. Indeed, Glogau and Kane observed bruising[5, 6] in up to 24% of their Restylane® and Perlane® patients and Tzikas[7] recorded 68% bruising in small sample of patients injected with Radiesse.®

12

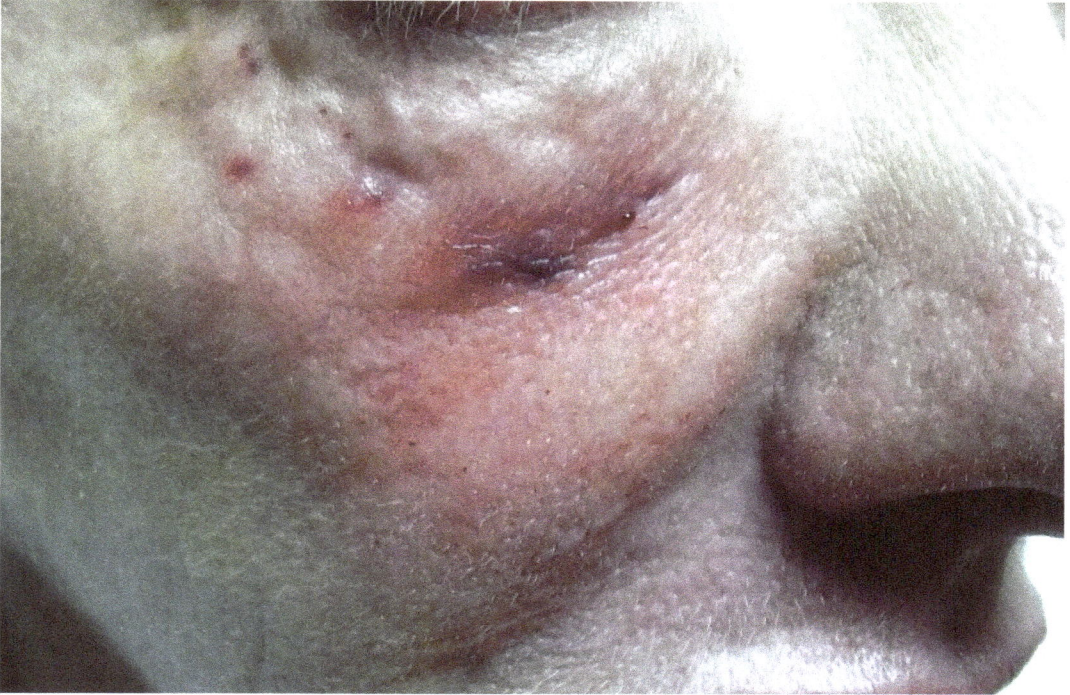

High Incidence of Bruising from Needle Injection of Cosmetic Wrinkle Fillers

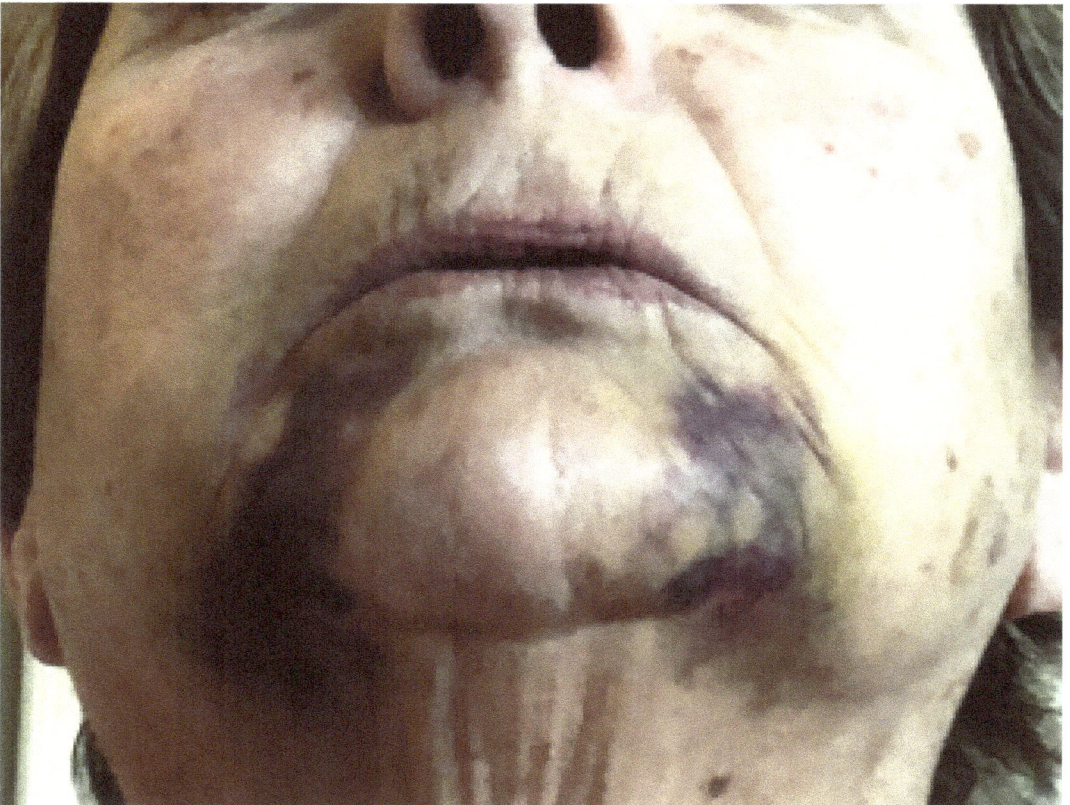

Marionette Line Bruising from HA Filler Hypodermic Needle Injection
by Las Vegas Plastic Surgeon

Consequently, it was revolutionary when attention abruptly shifted from product improvement to improving product delivery – from the sharp-tipped needle to the blunt-tipped microcannula.[8, 9] Instead of the traditional hypodermic needle, the microcannula is proving to be a safer way to inject cosmetic fillers...with less bruising, less swelling, and less pain.[10, 11, 12] Now we actually can inject wrinkles – without needles – so long as entry is introduced by a Pilot needle. In my practice, I estimate a 75% reduction in the use of needles – and their undesirable effects – because of our use of microcannula.

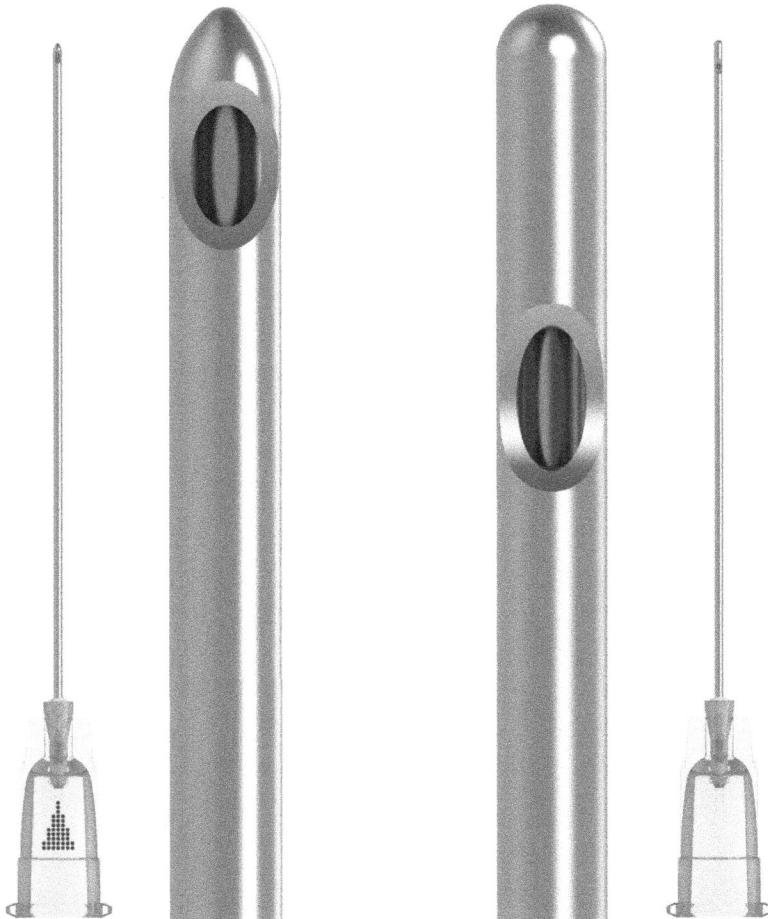

Moreover, the same patients who seek cosmetic injectable fillers for wrinkles also seek outpatient microneedling, laser, radio-frequency, or other energy treatments for skin rejuvenation, hair reduction, scar revision, skin-tightening, hyperpigmentation, and collagen stimulation. This is the reason for the genesis and rapid proliferation of the Medical Spa concept, which we began in Las Vegas & Henderson in 2001 – before the name Medical Spa was even coined – as perhaps the very first Medical Spa in the USA.

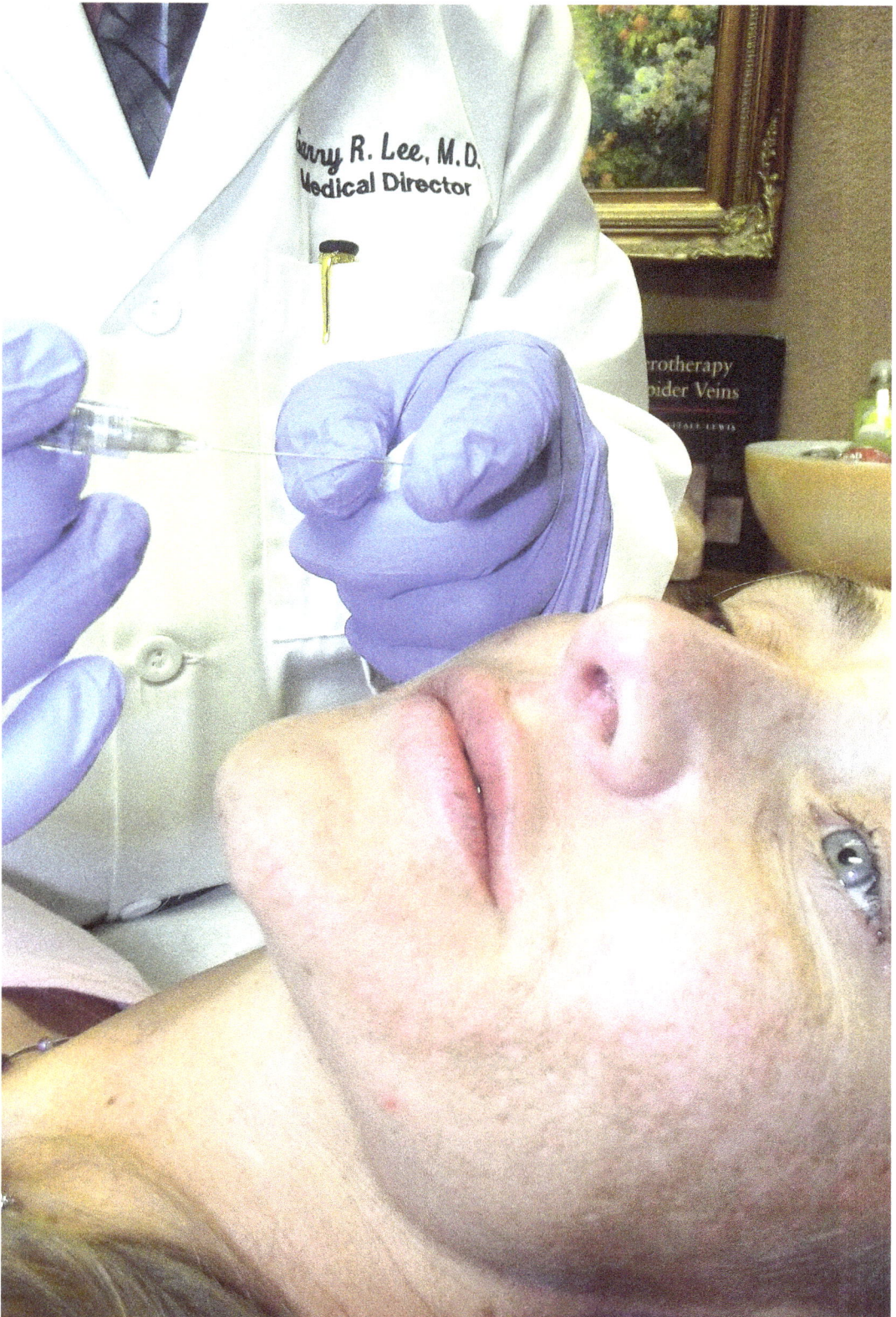

The Award Winning TSK STERiGLIDE Microcannula from Japan Has a Blunt & Tapered Tip

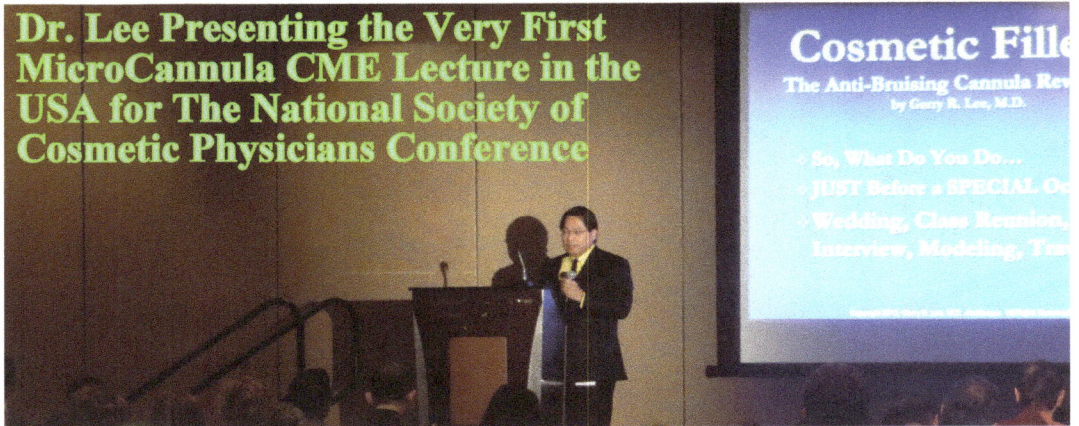

Lecturing for the National Society of Cosmetic Physicians, 2012

In 2012, I had the honor to present the first lecture to the National Society of Cosmetic Physicians in the USA on the use of microcannula for the injection of cosmetic wrinkle fillers – the first, I believe, to designate the microcannula "revolution.'" The challenge today is simply to discover the best ways to use microcannula as we progress from "revolution" to "evolution"…and now to what I term "convolution," or the optimal integration of multiple procedures to produce a synergy together.

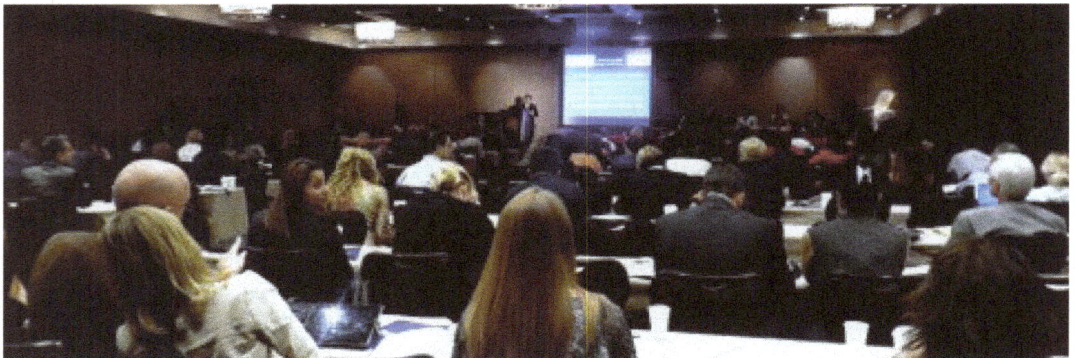

Dr. Lee's 2012 Lecture to the National Society of
Cosmetic Physicians on Advanced Injection Techniques.

The following microcannula cosmetic filler injection techniques described herein simply are the techniques I have originated in the USA; they are not definitive in nature, and are not a substitute for the critical experience of hands-on, personalized instruction to utilize these off-label applications safely. This book is an adjunct – not a replacement – for the sheer necessity of aesthetic preceptorship hands-on skills training by highly proficient clinical practitioners in this rapidly expanding non-invasive field.

What is an Aesthetic Microcannula?

A cannula[13] is "a small tube for insertion into a body cavity or into a duct or vessel," which originated circa 1684, derived from the Latin for "reed." Now commonly called microcannula, reflecting the size, aesthetic medicine usage is perhaps more precisely defined[14] as a "small tube with an edge that is not sharp, designed for atraumatic intradermal (or subdermal) injections…that can be used for the injection of cosmetic wrinkle fillers, like Hyaluronic Acid, Collagen, poly-L-lactic acid, CaHA, etc." Appearing much like the needle it replaces, the aesthetic microcannula markedly differs in that filler extrusion is only though a tiny opening, or extrusion port, near the blunt-end tip.

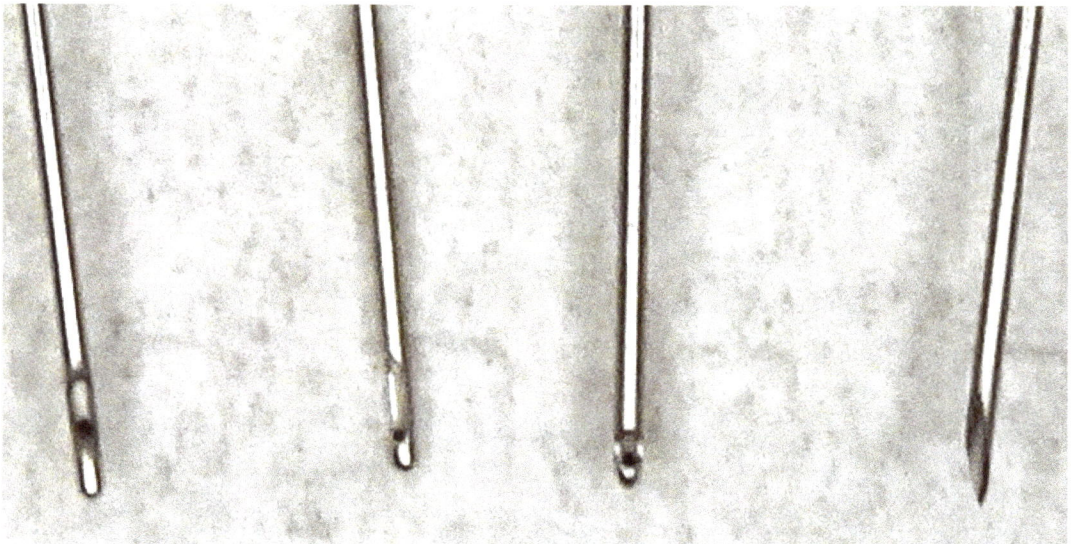

Microcannula (MC) from left:
DermaSculpt, Korean MC, TSK Steriglide MC; and 27 Gauge Needle

Safer; Less Pain, Swelling, & Bruising

Publications are scarce, but slowly accumulating, supporting the use of aesthetic microcannula over the traditional hypodermic needle. Niamtu[11] in 2009, and later in 2011,[12] reported less injection pain, less edema, and less bruising using fat injection cannula for cosmetic filler injections.

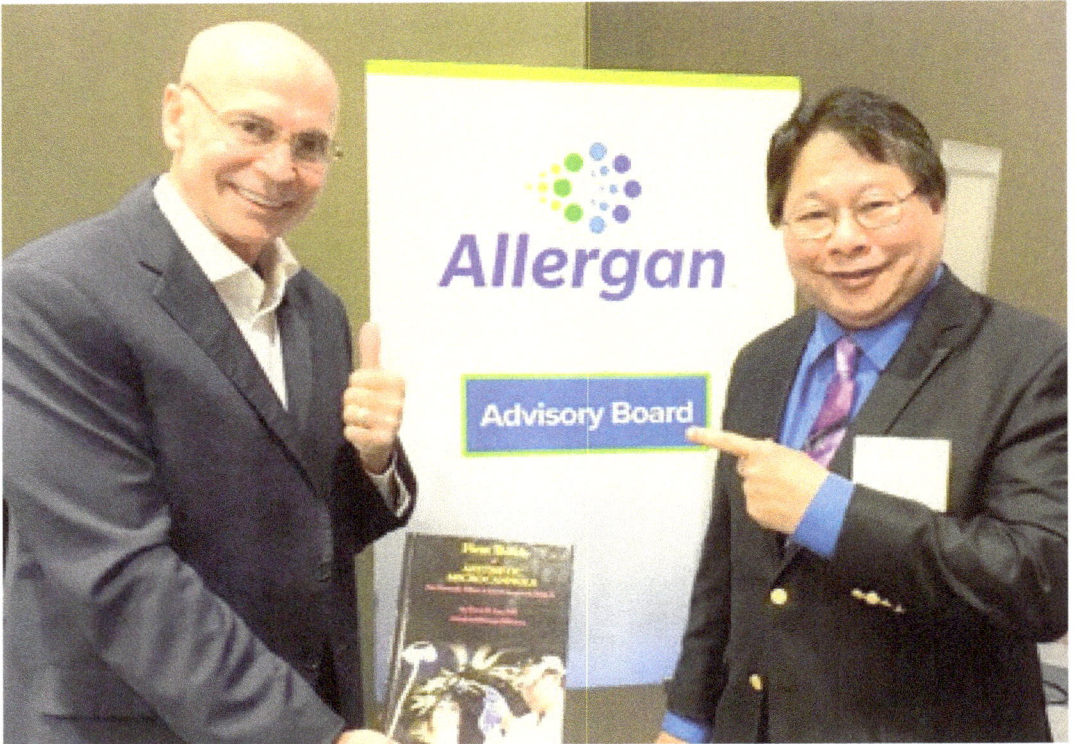

With Dr. Joe Niamtu at Allergan National Advisory Board Meeting

Fulton and Dewandre, et al[15] also noted less bruising, less ecchymosis, and less pain – which was quantified as 3 (mild) for injections with microcannula, increasing to 6 (moderate) with the hypodermic needle on a 10 point scale.

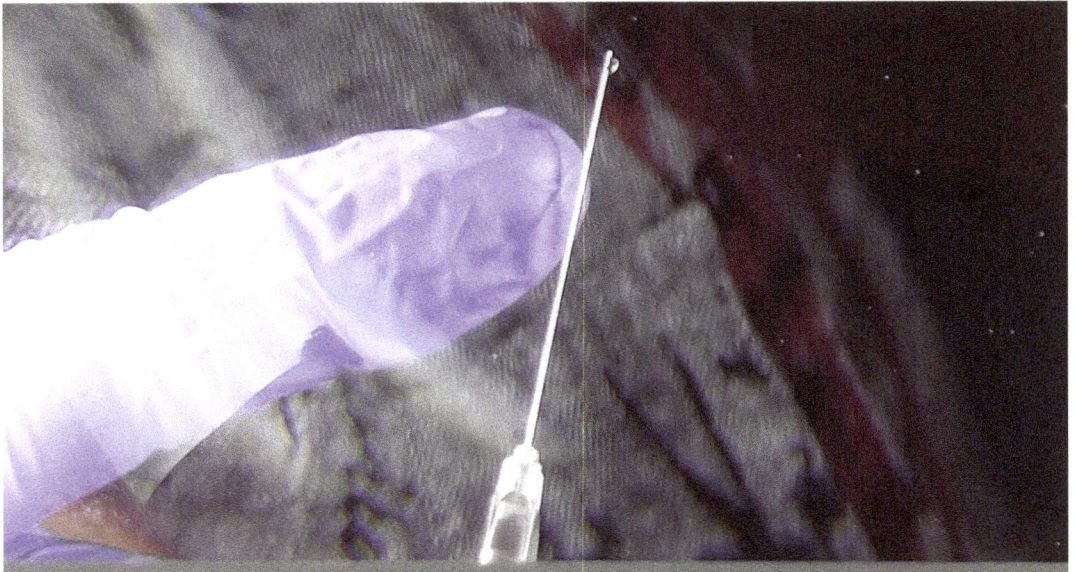

The TSK STERiGLIDE Microcannula with the Extrusion Port at the Tapered Blunt End Tip

They found no significant differences in a comparison of cosmetic filler results using the Global Aesthetic Improvements Scale Score between the hypodermic needle and the microcannula.

In 2012, Hexel et al[16] conducted a double-blind, randomized, controlled clinical trial to compare safety and efficacy of a metallic cannula with that of a standard needle for soft tissue augmentation of the nasolabial folds. Hexel concluded cannula were safe and useful to inject hyaluronic acid fillers into nasolabial folds with less pain, edema, hematoma, and redness than needles.

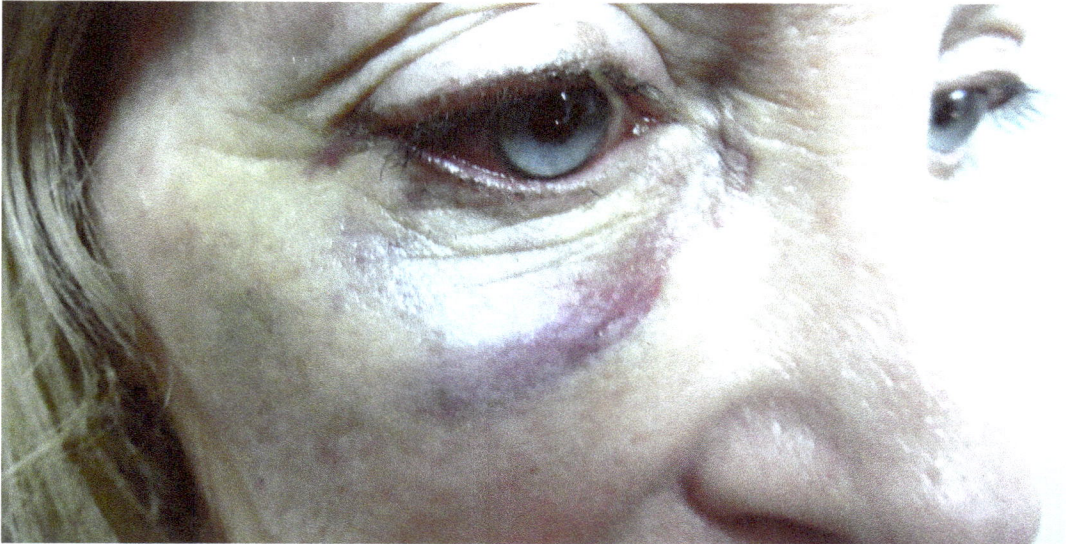

Tear Trough & Cheek Bruising After Cosmetic Injections

In 2012, Lazzeri et al[17] surveyed a total of 32 cases in 29 articles on permanent blindness from cosmetic filler injections. There were 15 cases after adipose injections and 17 non-adipose cases using corticosteroids, paraffin, silicone oil, collagen, polymethylmethacrylate, hyaluronic acid, and calcium hydroxyapatite. Lazzeri's prevention recommendation: to use microcannulas.

While it is incontrovertible that blunt-tip microcannulas are thought to be less likely to penetrate blood vessels and other tissue than sharp-tipped hypodermic needles, substantiating research is lacking.[18, 19] Of course, even a blunt tip does not ensure that one cannot penetrate any tissue – if one is forceful and aggressive enough – but safer tools are instrumental to producing better results. Nevertheless, a consensus is growing for the use of microcannula in conjunction with Pilot (or introducer) needles over the sole use of hypodermic needles.[20, 21]

Early pioneers used readily available larger gauge liposuction (non-disposable) metallic[11] cannulas designed for fat transfer, which required sterilization before re-use. However, particular care must be taken to carefully monitor the process to insure there is no risk of disease transmission. Hence, now that disposable microcannulas are affordable and readily available, our choice is always to use disposable microcannulas rather than to sterilize.

When NOT to Use Aesthetic Microcannula

Microcannulas are not recommended for fibrous scars, deep peri-oral vertical lines, the lip philtrum columns, Cupid's Bow, and if just one or two injections are needed. The sharp points of hypodermic needles are necessary to penetrate fibrous scars and to lift deep peri-oral lines. Of course, if just one or two injections are needed, it's easier and simpler to just use a hypodermic needle instead of using a Pilot needle and a microcannula.

Selection of Pilot Needle for Microcannula

The microcannula, being blunt tipped, is specifically designed not to penetrate blood vessels, nerves, and muscle, so a "Pilot" or introducer needle is necessary to create the opening through the skin. Of course, the larger the opening, the easier it is to insert the microcannula, but correspondingly, the greater trauma results in more pain, bruising, and swelling. On the other hand, the smaller the opening, the more difficult it is to insert the microcannula which can result in significant pain upon repeated attempts and failures at entry. Consequently, the ideal selection is dependent upon the dexterity of the individual injector to choose the smallest Pilot needle which rarely requires re-entry.

My usual choice is the 23 gauge ½" Pilot needle for the 27 gauge 1½" standard diameter microcannula for Juvederm,® Restylane,® and Belotero Balance,® or a difference of approximately 4 gauge sizes. In higher risk areas which require less precision, such as the cheek, I sometimes use a 25 gauge 1½" microcannula with a 21 gauge 1" Pilot needle since the blunter tip may be less likely to penetrate blood vessels.

Alternatively, when we use Sculptra,® we use larger diameter 25 gauge microcannula for facial treatments into the cheek and temporal fossa, and an even larger 22 gauge microcannula for cellulite and buttock shaping enhancements with a Pilot needle 4 gauge sizes larger. The larger diameter microcannula minimizes the inherent tendency of Sculptra® to clog in conjunction with the addition of additional dilution.

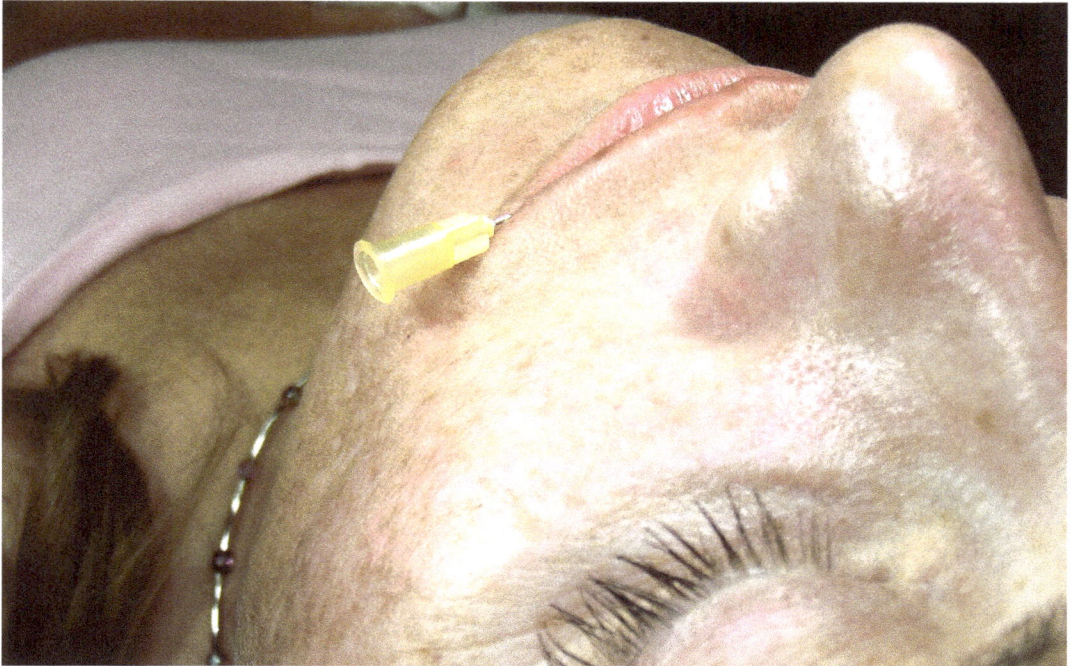

Pilot Needle Placement for Juvederm® Lip Enhancement

Insertion of Pilot Needle for Microcannula

I prefer to insert the Pilot needle at a 30° to 45° angle quickly into the superficial subcutaneous tissue just beneath the dermis in the direction I wish the microcannula to travel. Insertion too superficially will not penetrate the skin adequately and create difficulty in traversing the entry for the microcannula. Care must be taken that the angle and plane of insertion of the microcannula must match that of the Pilot needle or this will increase the likelihood of being unable to insert the microcannula because the temporary opening created is misaligned.

Again, it is more painful to repeatedly attempt to place the microcannula through too shallow or tiny a Pilot hole, rather than to just inject once with a hypodermic needle. Insertion too deeply will cause unnecessary trauma to tissue and may precipitate the very bruising we wish to avoid. Consequently, if the microcannula cannot be inserted by the 2nd or 3rd attempt, I recommend applying ice briefly, then re-applying the Pilot needle – a bit deeper – into exactly the same opening. We also leave the needle in place a few seconds to allow for hemostasis (credit: Kian Karimi, MD, FACS) and enough time for the needle to create a transitory channel through tissue to ease entry. I also suggest rotating or twisting the Pilot needle just prior to removal to enhance the temporary potential space created.

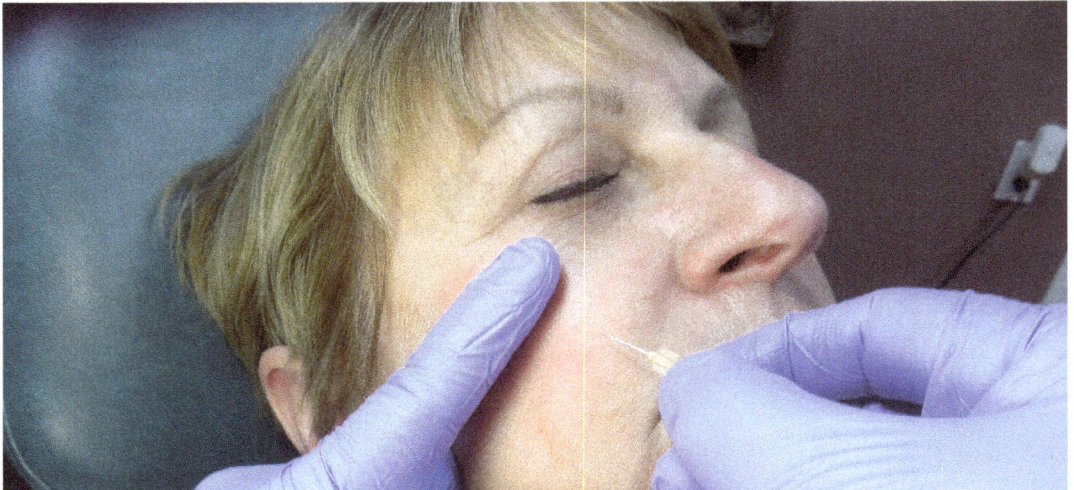

Selection of Disposable Microcannula

The differences are substantial in that some disposable microcannulas are so flexible, you cannot place cosmetic filler precisely where desired, and others are so rigid, you increase the likelihood of penetrating blood vessels as well as increasing the resulting pain. More importantly, the tip of the microcannula is vital in your ability to perform a smooth entry, in that a tapered tip is easier to place than one which is rounded and blunt. The other point to make is that the tip is best tapered for easier entry, but must not be too pointed that it facilitates entry into blood vessels or is at risk for breakage if weakened structurally. In our practice, I have never had a tip break from any reputable brand after thousands of uses over the years.

The other critical issue in the differentiation of microcannulas is the placement of the extrusion port or opening at the end of the microcannula. Ideally, the extrusion port should be as near as possible to the tip to more precisely place the cosmetic filler product exactly where intended. For example, if I wish to inject the most lateral corner of the lip, I don't want the filler to be extruded so medial that I have to attempt to massage it into the intended corner. See the photographs below to compare the relative distances between the extrusion port and the tip of the most popular brands in the USA.

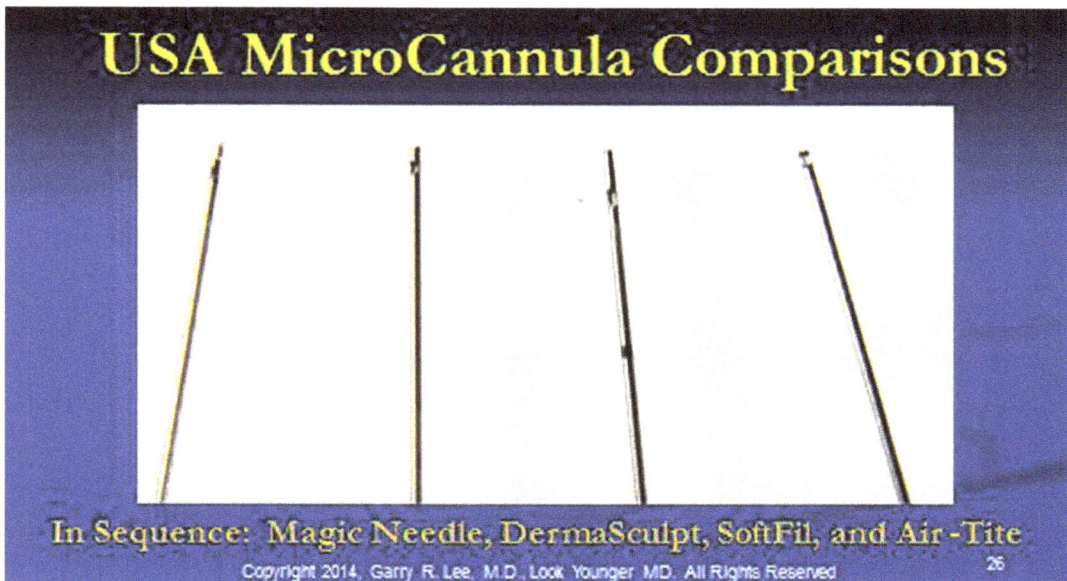

USA MicroCannula Comparisons

In Sequence: Magic Needle, DermaSculpt, SoftFil, and Air-Tite

Copyright 2014, Garry R. Lee, M.D., Look Younger MD. All Rights Reserved

Comparison of Extrusion Ports Showing Distance from Tip and Variable Tip Tapering

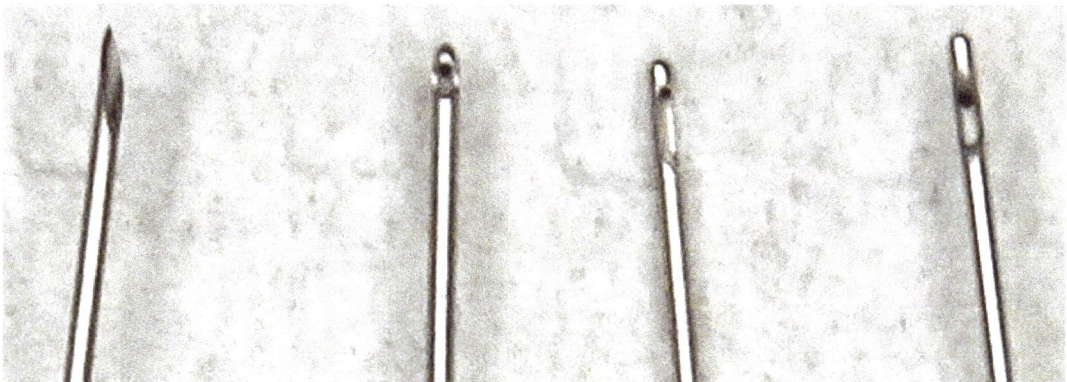

In Sequence: 27 Gauge Needle and microcannula: Japanese TSK STERiGLIDE, Korean, and French DermaSculpt

Another salient issue is the selection of the gauge and length of the microcannula. Microcannulas may be used with nearly every type of cosmetic filler, but the nature of the filler will direct the size of the microcannula. Typically, I match the size of the microcannula to the gauge of the cosmetic filler's recommended needle. If difficult to extrude, I simply select a larger diameter microcannula. If there is too much entry trauma, bruising, or pain, I select a smaller diameter microcannula and corresponding Pilot needle, but take extra care not to inject too forcefully or too quickly to over-stress the hub's original design parameters. Forcing cosmetic filler into a smaller gauge microcannula than its original design can rupture the hub of the syringe.

Another consideration is for those who dilute their cosmetic filler differently so that the viscosity of the filler is changed. For example, the amount of sterile water and local anesthetic used in each Sculptra® bottle varies widely by different practitioners when injected into the temple. This results in vast differences in the apparent "lumpiness" in this thin-skinned area and the degree of Sculptra® clogging within the microcannula shaft. Consequently, each practitioner must adjust the size of the microcannula to accommodate differences in viscosity.

Microcannula length is dictated by the need for enough rigidity to precisely place the cosmetic filler where desired, but with enough flexibility to tunnel gently around obstructions or to find or to create the potential channel we are seeking. In general, I personally find the 2" microcannulas too flexible and the 1" microcannulas too short to get into most places; consequently, I typically use 27 gauge 1½" TSK STERiGLIDE microcannulas. The TSK STERiGLIDE aesthetic microcannula, designed for nearest-to-tip precision filler delivery, is manufactured in Japan and distributed in the USA by Air-Tite.

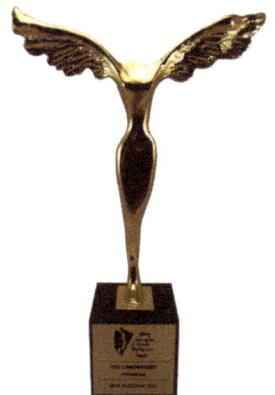

The TSK STERiGLIDE Microcannula won the Prestigious
International Anti-Aging & Beauty Trophy for Best Injection Tool Over Other Microcannula

Selection of Cosmetic Filler

My primary cosmetic injectable filler of choice is currently hyaluronic acid (HA), such as Juvederm® (Allergan) or Restylane® (Galderma), because any imperfection can easily be remedied with the enzyme, hyaluronidase.[22, 64, 65]   I use Juvederm Ultra Plus XC® almost everywhere because I want a cosmetic injectable filler that I can dissolve almost instantly if I accidentally inject into a blood vessel, and clinically, I believe it may last a little longer than Restylane.®

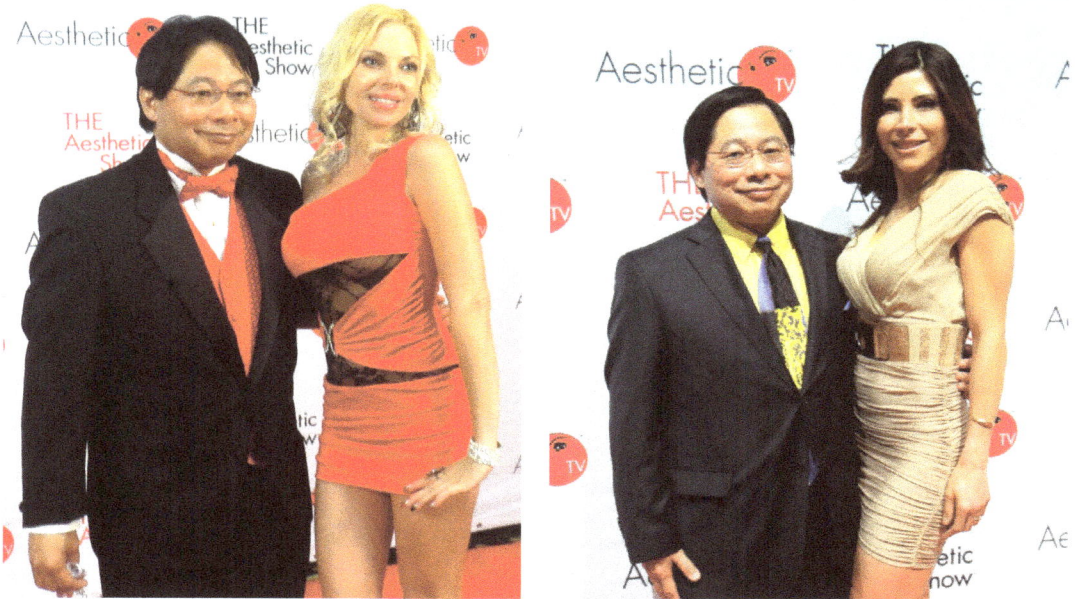

Cosmetic Injection Patient Models: Beverly Willett & Gaby Dominguez – The Aesthetic Awards

Indeed, in 2018, The American Society for Aesthetic Plastic Surgery[23] noted that hyaluronic acid fillers constituted an astounding 93.1% of all injectable fillers in the USA, or 810,240 of a total of 870,097 procedures.

Two exceptions in 2019 are under the eyes in the Tear Trough, where I use Mertz's Belotero Balance® because it appears to cause less swelling; and Restylane Lyft® supra-periosteal in the cheek or Zygomatic arch, because it is effective yet less costly than Juvederm Voluma® and there are fewer reports of nodule formation with it. I avoid the use of long lasting or "permanent" fillers which cannot be modified without the need for surgical excision and the resulting risk of scar formation.[24]

Nevertheless, I suggest physicians consider all of the comparable products on the market before arriving upon your individual selection. I occasionally use other fillers if they possess special properties to stimulate native production of collagen, such as Radiesse® for the dorsum of hands, and Sculptra® in the temple and buttocks for contouring and cellulite.

Other physicians use autologous fat harvested from liposuction in larger diameter microcannula, or cannula, using similar techniques, but which can be unpredictable and irregular in degree of survival after placement.[25] Inconsistent fat survival often causes a "lumpy" aspect in appearance such as the example below, which I had to correct using HA fillers.

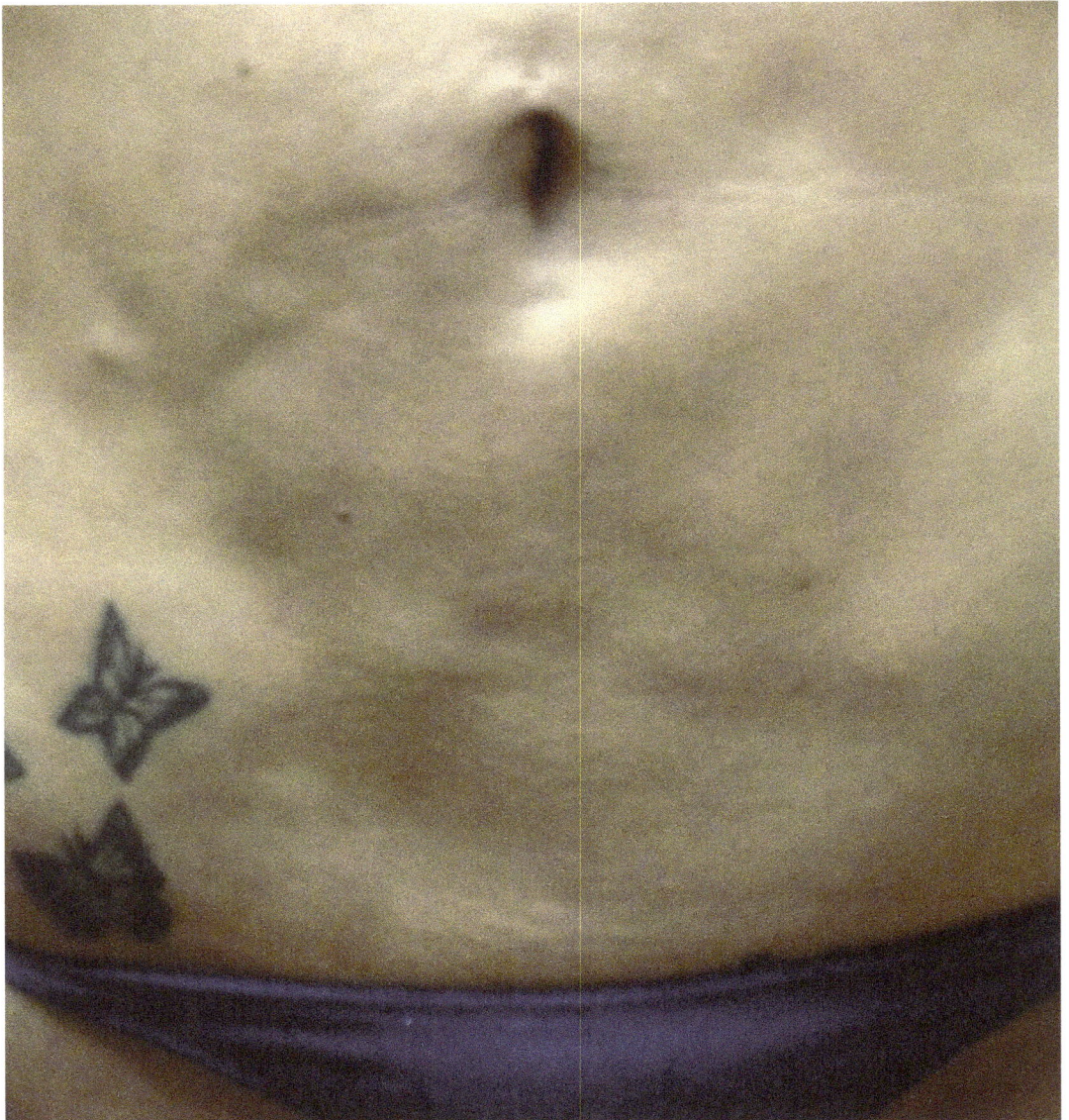

Irregular (Patchy) Autologous Fat Survival After Fat Abdominal Injection

Basic Facial Anatomy
for Filler Injections

Of course it is critical to know the anatomy of the area you are treating to know where to inject – and in particular, where NOT to inject – regardless of whether it is with a hypodermic needle or a microcannula. Consequently, the following illustrations identify some of the major anatomical landmarks which must be navigated in order to avoid the most hazardous areas for injection. The cardinal risk, of course, is inadvertently injecting into a blood vessel, resulting in necrosis[26] of the areas distal to blockage, or even embolization of cosmetic injectable filler resulting in catastrophic sequelae, such as tissue infarction, stroke, or blindness.[34]

Again, this book is designed for the clinical practitioner rather than the academic researcher or medical school instructor, so the most commonly encountered hazards are highlighted for your clinical correlation rather than minutiae, which focuses upon the least relevant.

Critically important is the realization that any generic anatomical diagram is only a generalization of the actuality of the specific anatomy of each individual patient; hence we must always keep in mind that there are significant variants to the location of each structure naturally, and especially after scar formation from trauma or surgical intervention in the injected area. Consequently, any diagram is only an approximate guide to where any particular structure usually is – rather than a certainty of where it must be.

The evolution of technique in 2019 is in injecting cosmetic fillers more precisely using the actual changes in the anatomy of how we age to treat wrinkles. In the past, we merely used the superficial contours of the skin in replacing the lost volume of subcutaneous fat and other tissue. This is can be effective, but I believe the better technique is to replace what we have lost… precisely where we have lost it.

Clinically, this means that we have now changed our approach, especially in the cheek, to address the underlying atrophy of the Deep Medial and Lateral

Cheek Fat compartments first, since we are now aware that this selective loss of foundation[27, 48] is a primary cause of the superficial appearance of the aging face. Moreover, a current concept is that the collapse of the deep fat compartment causes the superficial fat compartment to slide downwards in response to gravity and hence the injection of cosmetic filler in the superficial compartments will only give rise to a distorted reconstruction of the patient's natural appearance. In other words, only refilling the structure above does not reconstruct the loss of the foundation below.

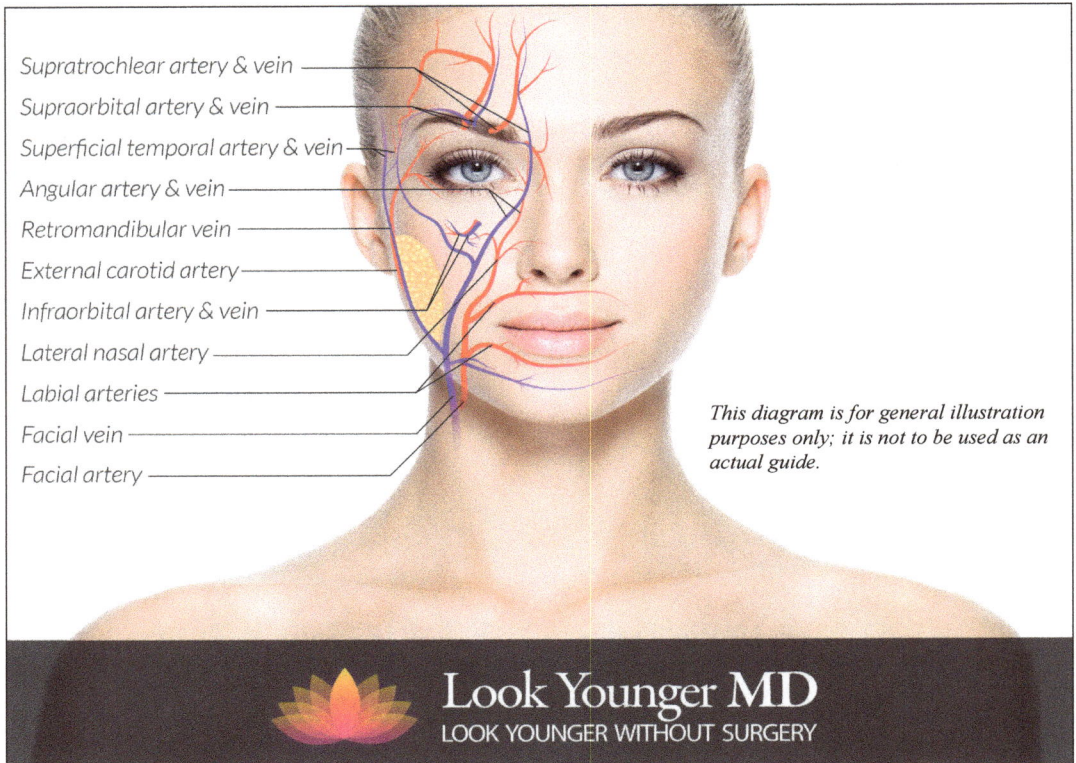

Supratrochlear artery & vein
Supraorbital artery & vein
Superficial temporal artery & vein
Angular artery & vein
Retromandibular vein
External carotid artery
Infraorbital artery & vein
Lateral nasal artery
Labial arteries
Facial vein
Facial artery

This diagram is for general illustration purposes only; it is not to be used as an actual guide.

Look Younger **MD**
LOOK YOUNGER WITHOUT SURGERY

The next question is how best to replace this selective loss of midface foundation since there are many effective approaches by many highly respected practitioners.

Cheek Technique

Our cheek approach is to use the AccuVein™ [29] to mark the major blood vessels in this area beforehand and then insert the Pilot needle into the relatively avascular area lateral to the ala of the nose, just lateral to where it intersects the mid-pupillary line. We inject the Pilot needle aiming deep – not into the dermal-SQ junction – directly at the most medial superior aspect of the Deep Medial

Cheek Fat. We then tunnel in slowly and gently with the microcannula using the "Wiggle Progression" Technique (page 40) we presented in 2012, whereby we advance ever so slowly forward constantly asking the patient to indicate the slightest discomfort, or alternatively, if we can "feel" a slight obstruction to advancement. This is analogous to using any patient discomfort at all as an early warning navigation probe through the sea of potential anatomical hazards which the blunt tip of the microcannula can signal to us before inducing any significant trauma.

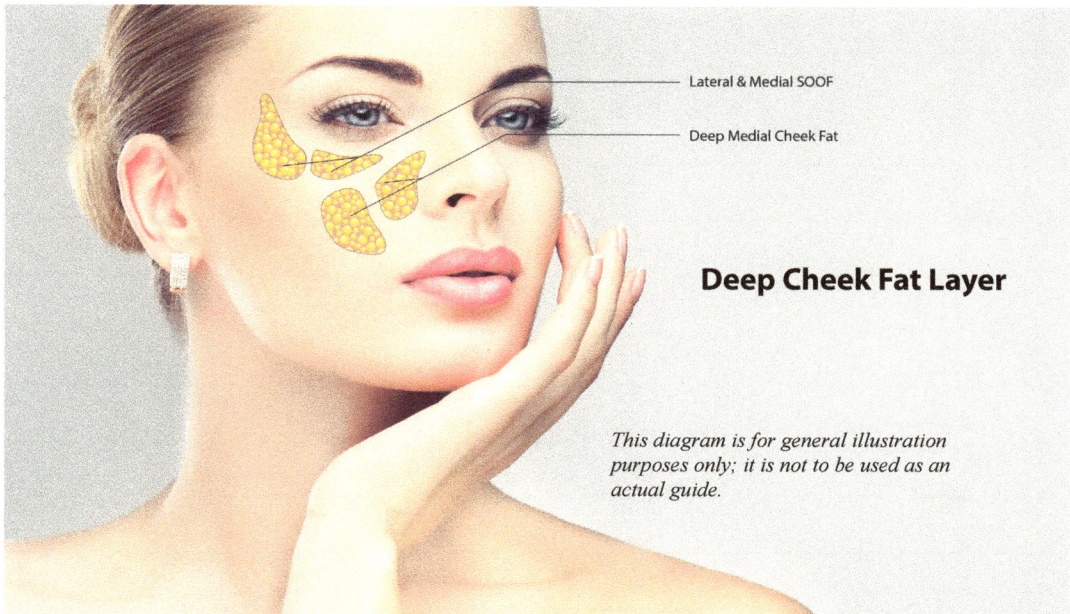

Lateral & Medial SOOF

Deep Medial Cheek Fat

Deep Cheek Fat Layer

This diagram is for general illustration purposes only; it is not to be used as an actual guide.

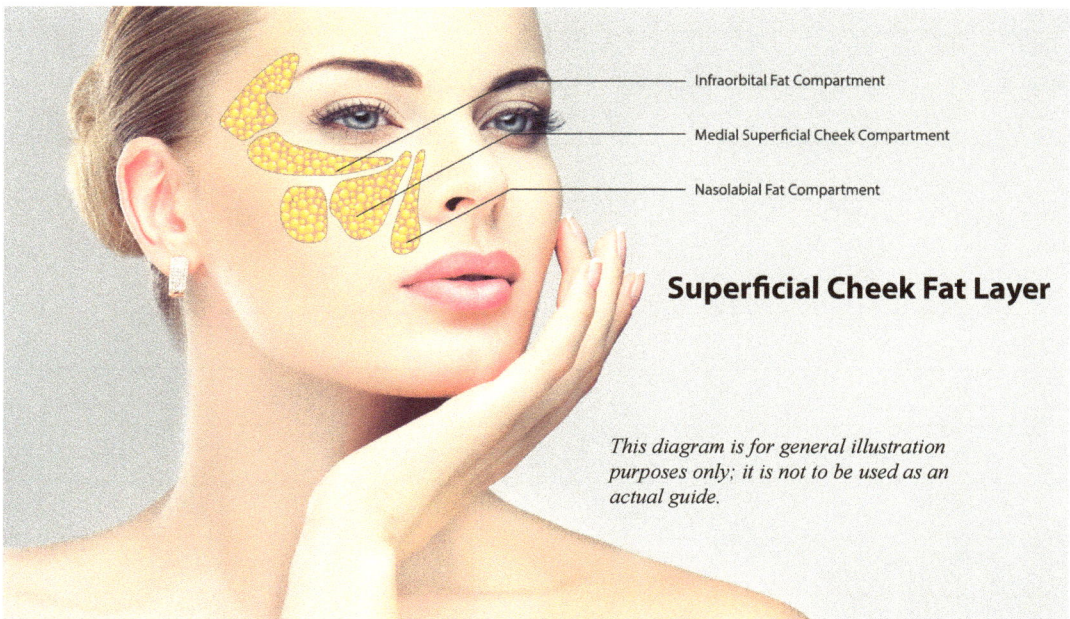

Infraorbital Fat Compartment

Medial Superficial Cheek Compartment

Nasolabial Fat Compartment

Superficial Cheek Fat Layer

This diagram is for general illustration purposes only; it is not to be used as an actual guide.

NOTES

Basic Microcannula Facial Techniques

〜〜〜

Skin Cleansing, Numbing, & Aseptic Protocol

Hibiclens and isopropyl alcohol (70%) has long been the topical cleansing agents used prior to the injection of cosmetic wrinkle fillers, however, the increasing concern that the use of Hibiclens[30] is contraindicated around the eyes has led us to the search for better agents, particularly as our current injection depth is periosteal in the cheek and temporal fossa increasing the risk of osteomyelitis. Moreover, the increasing concern over the risk of biofilm from a nidus of infection also propelled the search for a better agent than that of just alcohol alone.

Upon the recommendation of Dermatologist Patrick Bitter, Jr., we have shifted our cleansing protocol predominately to the use of hypochlorous acid (0.009%, Lasercyn[31, 32]) which is economical enough for use in the cheek and temporal areas without the contraindication of Hibiclens. Remarkably, it is even effective for HIV and MRSA and lacks the stinging sensation and smell of the use of topical alcohol.

Of course, we all know that needle or microcannula filler injection is an aseptic – and not a sterile – procedure, nevertheless, we want to do our best to minimize the risk for cellulitis and osteomyelitis by the best protocols. Consequently, I now recommend an initial cleansing with topical alcohol adequate to remove any make-up present, followed by a topical spray of hypochlorous acid particularly in the cheek and temporal fossa.

I also use the TSK needle holder, place topical alcohol into it, and use it as the holder for my Pilot needle for maximal effect. I also keep the tip of the microcannula elevated on the rim of the sterile plastic filler container to minimize contact with the Mayo tray.

Skin Traction, Depth of Injection, & Aspiration

Inadequate traction is where most beginning microcannula users often fail. They fail to retract the skin adequately to insert the Pilot needle and the blunt tip repeatedly snags on loose skin at attempted entry, causing more pain than if a needle were used. Proficiency here is merely a matter of method and practice.

The original technique I use, described in our 2013 instructional video,[33] is simply to create enough skin tension to promote optimal resistance for entry in the direction of the insertion. I typically place traction in the direction opposite of the direction I am injecting the microcannula, a technique I call "opposing traction," which prevents loose skin from snagging the tip of the microcannula. The exception is in lips, where I often pull the lip into the direction in which I want the microcannula to travel to facilitate the opening of a potential entry channel, a microcannula technique I call "advancing traction." I think of it as a collapsed accordion which is much easier to transect when it is not collapsed onto itself.

Originally, we were trained to inject into the mid to deep dermis for cosmetic filler placement. With microcannula, however, the placement depends upon the cosmetic filler chosen and ranges from the dermal-subcutaneous (dermal-SQ) junction for most hyaluronic acid fillers to supra-periosteal for Juvederm Voluma® and Restylane Lyft.® I have yet to notice a significant change in the duration of action of any given filler by placement in the dermal-SQ junction instead of the dermis itself and am unaware of any current research to this effect.

Depth adjustment must also be made automatically to be deep enough to hide the appearance of lumpiness and to adjust for the natural anatomical variations of skin thickness by location, gender, and with aging. Placement must be deeper in older patients with thinner skin, especially in natural areas of thinness such as the temples and the Tear Trough. My observation is that the deeper the filler placement – the more volume you need – and that less product is required with more superficial placement to correct wrinkles.

I am a proponent of injection as we withdraw the microcannula in retrograde, because I believe we can find or create a potential space through subcutaneous tissue with microcannula using the Wiggle Progression Technique (described later). Consequently, injection as we are attempting to locate a potential space under the dermis is higher risk than injection once we know a potential space has actually been located.

Finally, the question remains on whether or not to aspirate with the microcannula in attempting to obtain a back-flash of blood in the hub of the syringe, indicative of injection into a blood vessel. Aspiration would allow us the opportunity of repositioning the tip of the microcannula out of a blood vessel, preventing accidental filler injection.

Anecdotally, we have had reports of success with aspiration; however recent research has clarified the difficulty of successfully aspirating blood in vivo clinical conditions. Our belief has been that it can do no harm as an additional safety procedure, and may indeed help, so we will continue to aspirate.[35, 36, 37, 38]

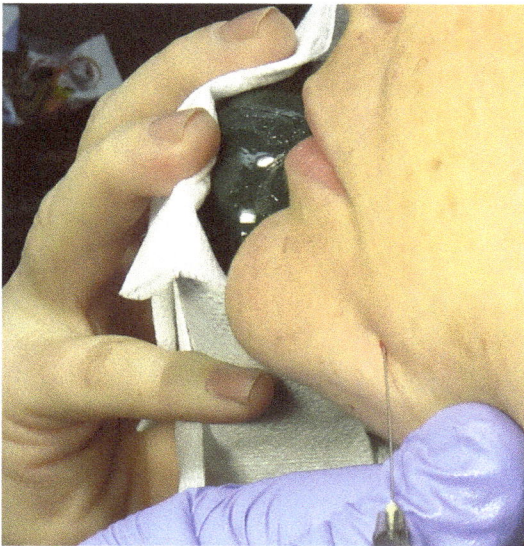

The Opposing Traction Technique in the Marionette Line Pulling in the Opposite Direction of Injection

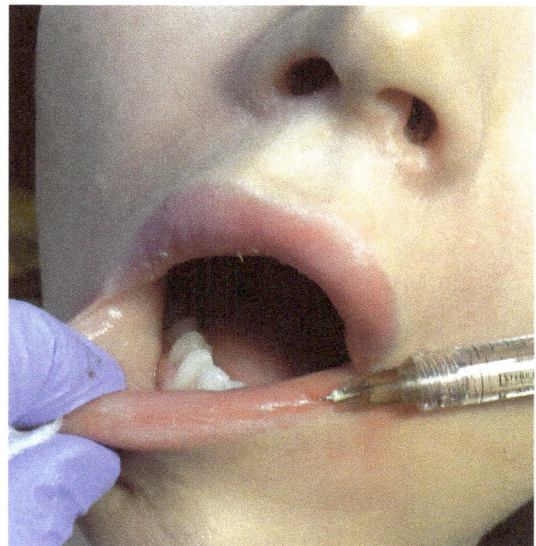

The Advancing Traction Lip Technique Pulling In the Direction of Injection

Long Microcannula Double Cross-Hatched Fan (LeeXX) Technique

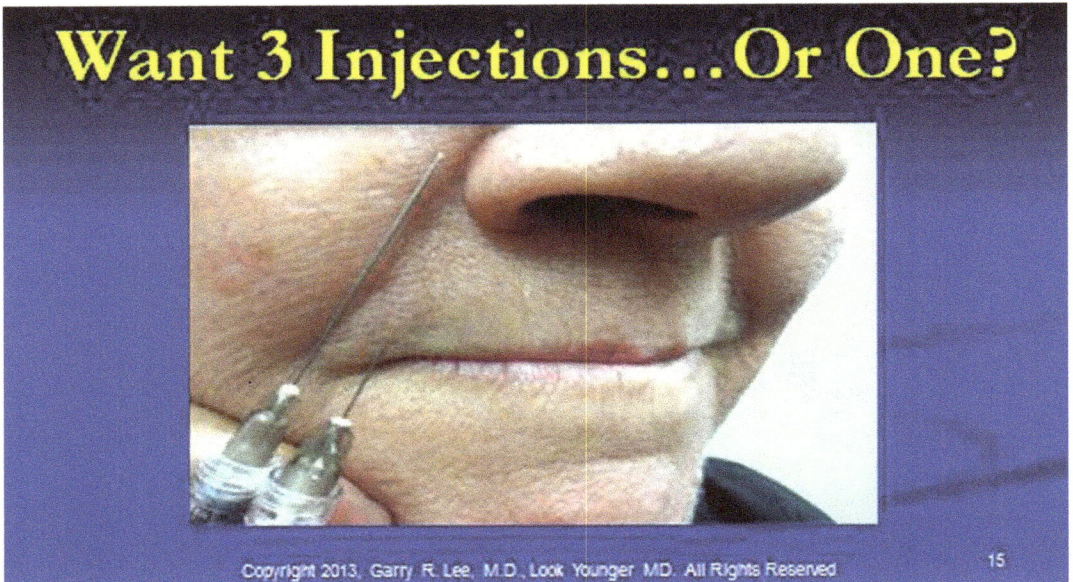

Allergan Packaged Needle Needs 3 Injections to Traverse Most Nasolabial Folds

When I first began teaching physicians, physician assistants, and nurses, I observed that the short ½" needles included with Juvederm® syringes required three traumatic needle insertions to encompass the length of the typical nasolabial fold. I was able to get the same results simply by replacing the ½" needle with the longer 1½" needle – with only one painful injection instead of three.

Then, when the microcannula obtained FDA Approval and became available in the USA, I simply replaced the 1½" needle with the 1½" microcannula. As I was seeking the best way to use microcannula, I wanted the least amount of needle trauma for the smoothest and most natural appearing results.

Consequently, I applied the basic fan technique whereby a single point of entry is made at the base of the nasolabial fold and aimed the microcannula superiorly into the nasolabial fold, injecting retrograde back to the point of entry – without removing the tip of the microcannula. Then, the fan was repeated medially and laterally from this baseline to span the entire nasolabial fold.

However, I truly wanted a cross-hatching effect for a more natural appearance and perhaps more longevity, so I bisected the nasolabial fold at right angles and repeated the process whereby the two fans would intersect with the addition of only one other Pilot hole, giving us "The Long Microcannula Double Cross-Hatched Fan Technique (LeeXX[19])." This same technique is adoptable to many other areas, but we use it almost exclusively in the nasolabial folds, the marionette lines, the submalar areas, and many body applications.

The Nasolabial Fold Technique (using LeeXX)

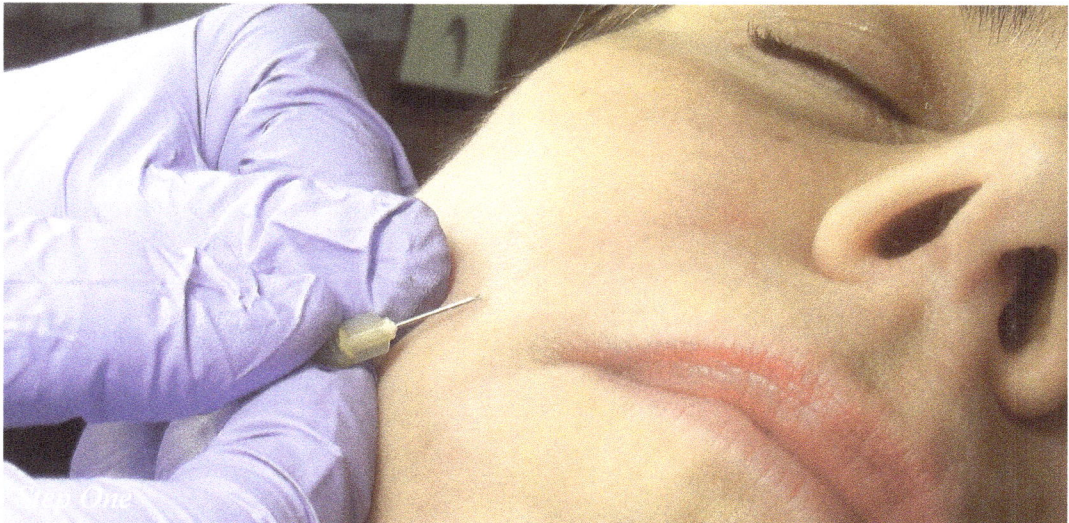

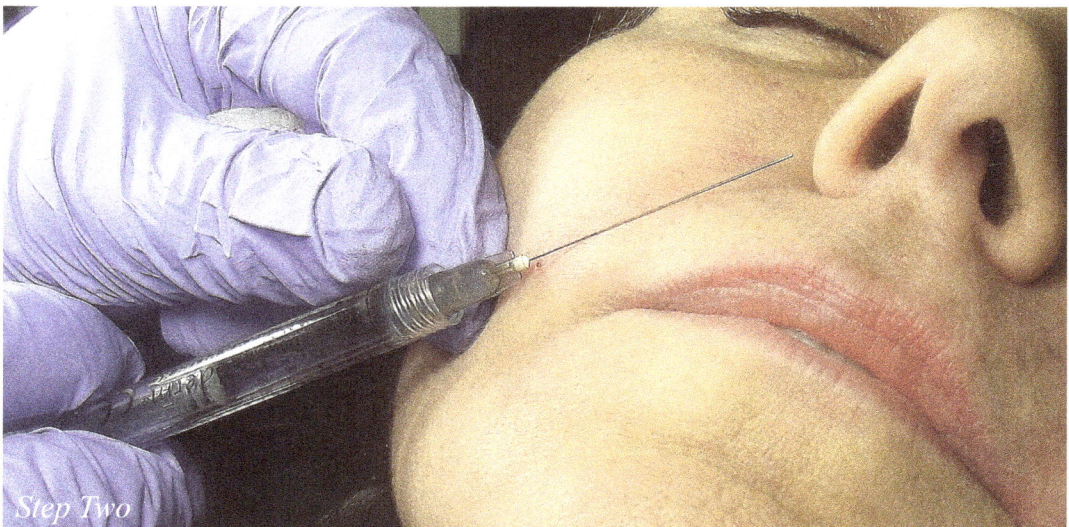

Long Microcannula Double Cross-Hatched Fan, Published September 2012, MedEsthetics

Step Three

Step Four

Step Five

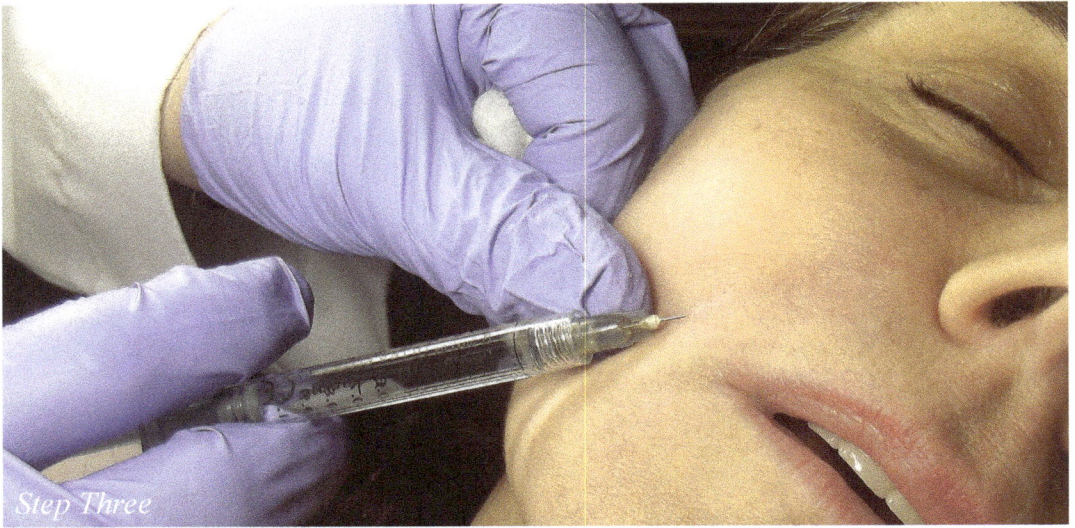

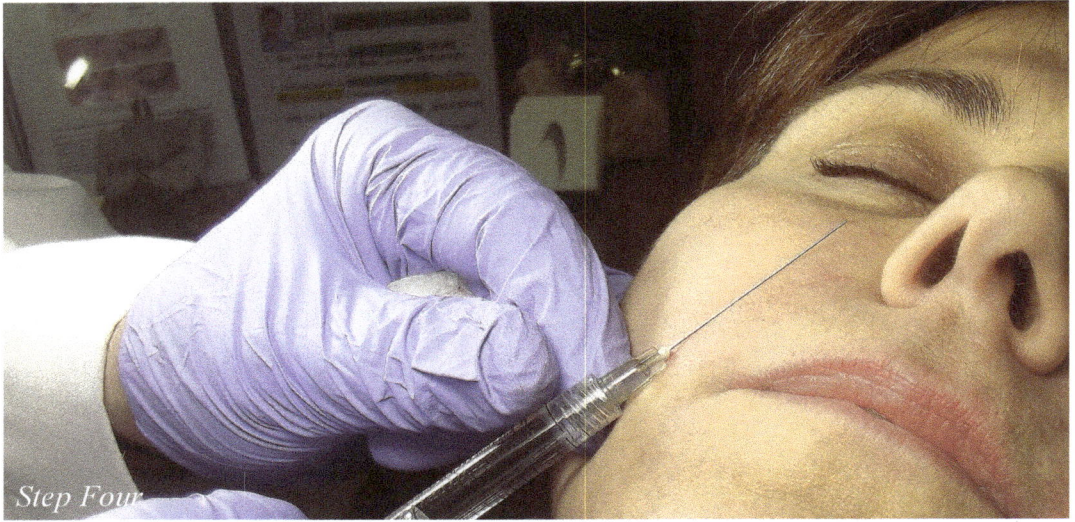

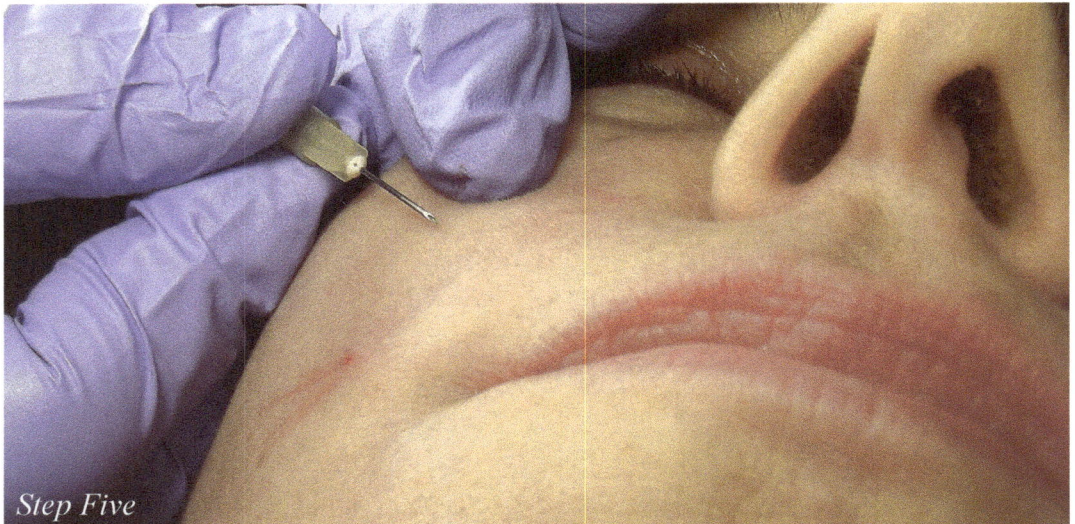

Long Microcannula Double Cross-Hatched Fan, Published September 2012, MedEsthetics

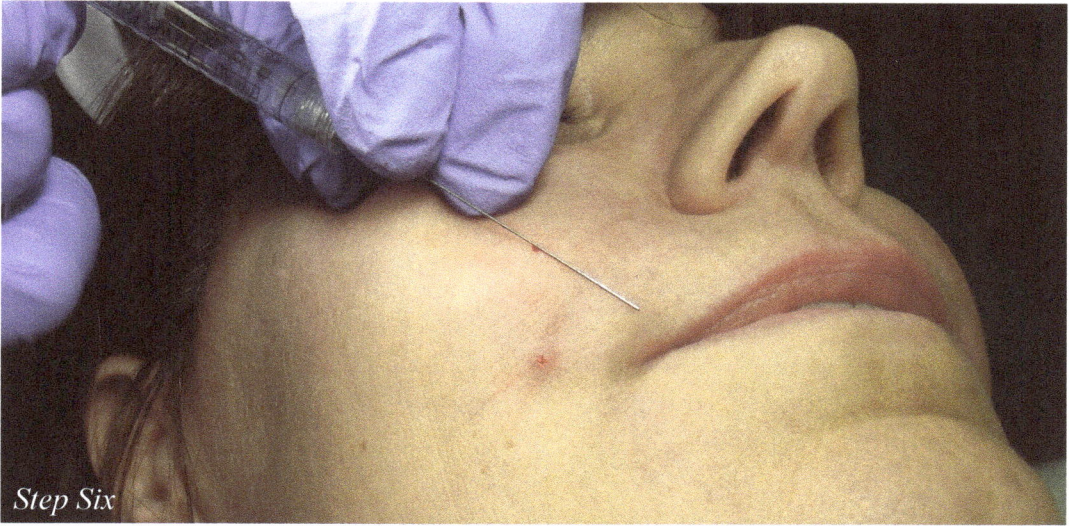

Step Six

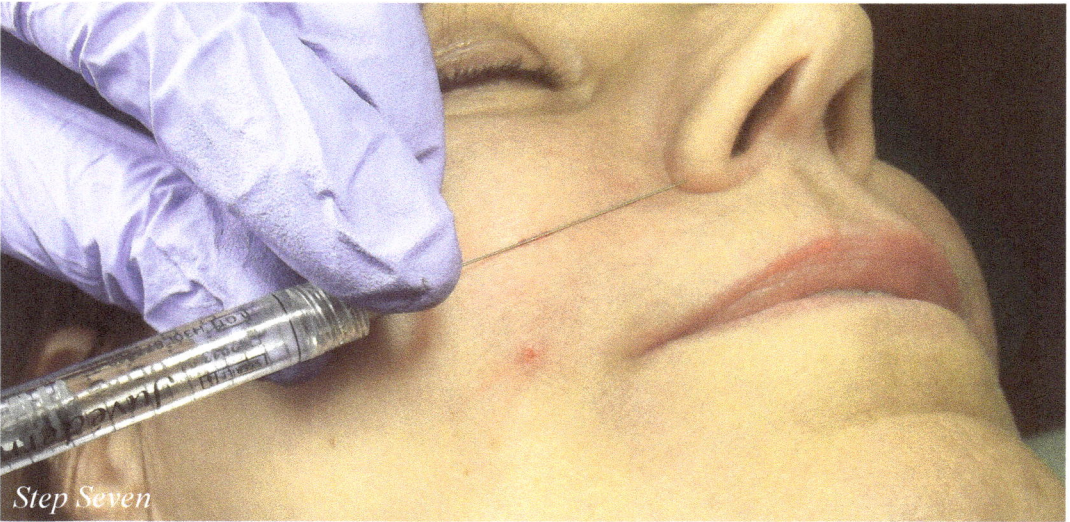

Step Seven

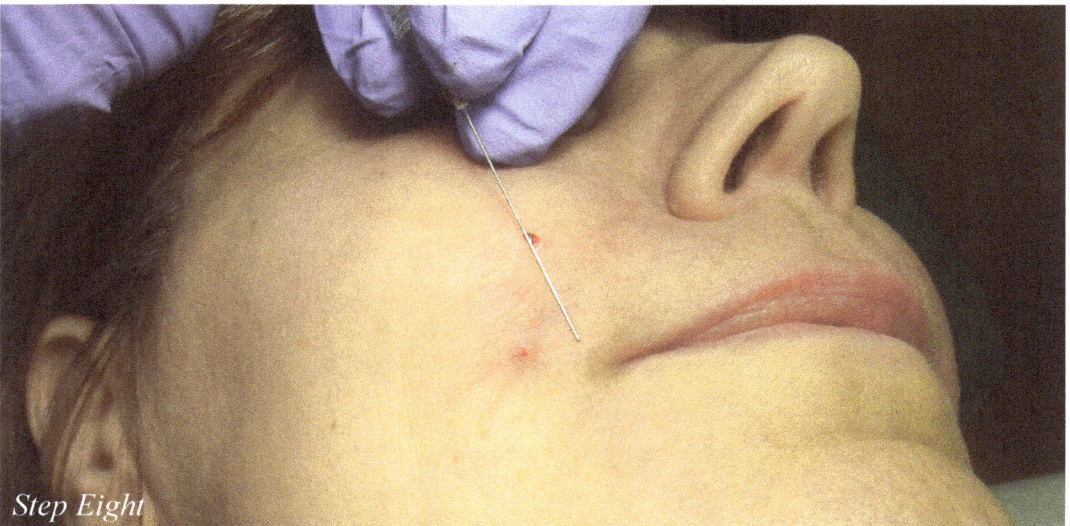

Step Eight

Long Microcannula Double Cross-Hatched Fan, Published September 2012, MedEsthetics

Marionette Technique

Often, the marionette line will have the shape of a check-mark with the smaller arm extending medially towards the chin. Just as the technique with the nasolabial fold, The Long Microcannula Double Cross-Hatched Fan Technique (LeeXX) is applied to the marionette line by placement of the Pilot needle into the inferior lateral aspect – the angle of the check-mark – and directing it upwards towards the corner of the mouth. After the first Pilot needle is removed, just replace it with the microcannula, fanning it medial and lateral to with enough retrograde injection of the chosen filler for approximately 90% correction of the marionette line.

The amount of absorption of water by each particular cosmetic injectable filler is dependent upon how relatively hydrophilic it is and the amount of swelling is dependent upon the amount of physical trauma to tissue during the injection process. Consequently, I typically under-fill slightly to accommodate for the expected degree of swelling. Overfill of the marionette line can cause a distortion of the natural anatomy much like the appearance of a chipmunk.

This analogy is usually used to describe the enlargement of the parotid gland, but in application to microcannula (MC) over-fill, I call it the ***Chipmunk Effect.***

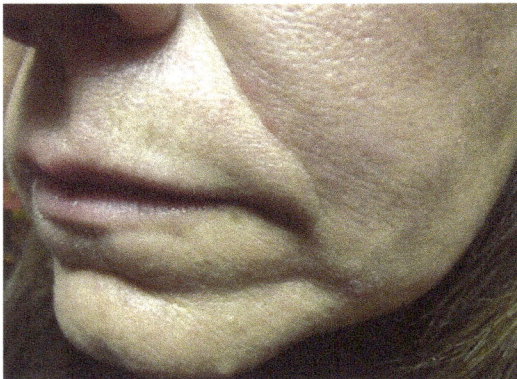

The MC Marionette Checkmark Sign

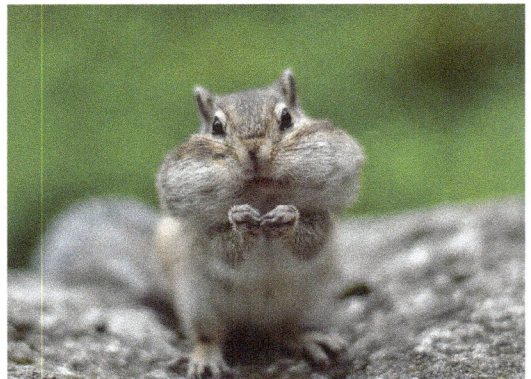

Excessive ML Fill May Cause the MC Chipmunk Effect

One of the pitfalls of the marionette line is that 100% correction usually is not possible when only treating this area in isolation. Often 30% or more of this apparent defect is due to the overlying skin above and lateral to it from volume loss in the cheek, so I usually caution the patient that only a partial correction is possible unless they also correct the volume loss from above.

Again, as in the nasolabial folds, I place the second Pilot needle at right angles to the first using The Long Microcannula Double Cross-Hatched Fan Technique (LeeXX) as well as the Wiggle Progression Technique (described next) to minimize any trauma to the area injected as well as to minimize the risk of accidentally injecting into a blood vessel.

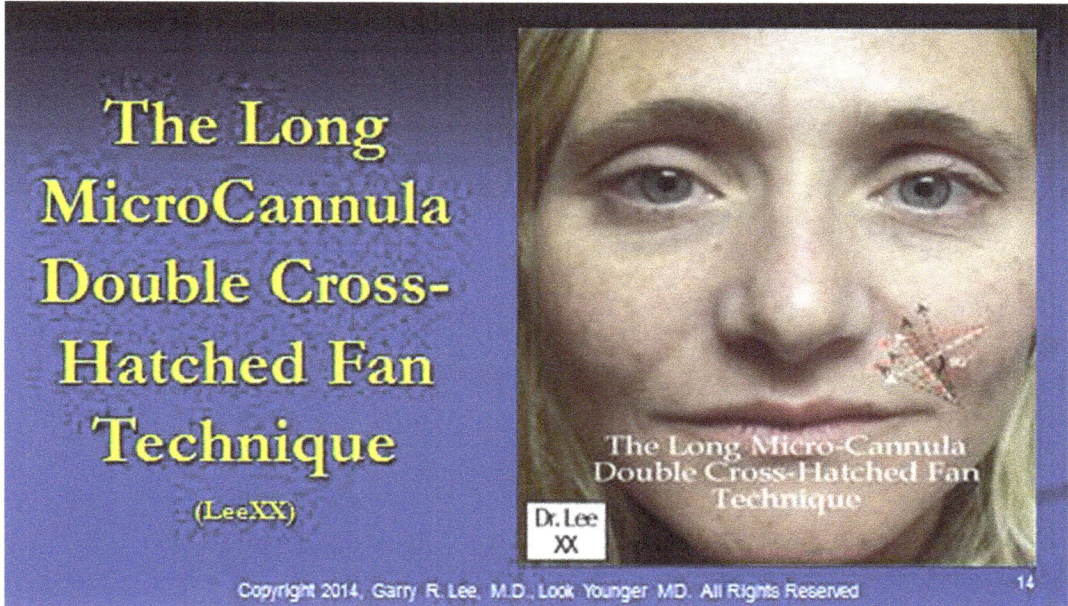

The Long MicroCannula Double Cross-Hatched Fan Technique

(LeeXX)

The Long Micro-Cannula Double Cross-Hatched Fan Technique

Dr. Lee XX

14

The Entire Nasolabial Fold Can Be Encompassed with Only 2 Pilot Holes Using This Technique

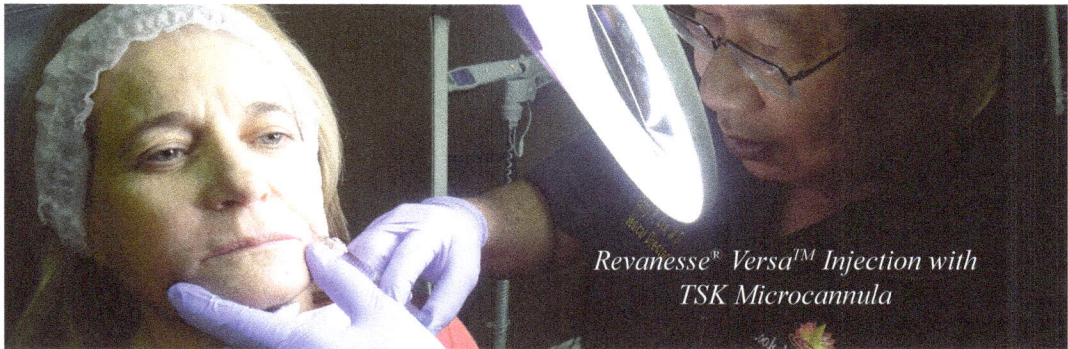

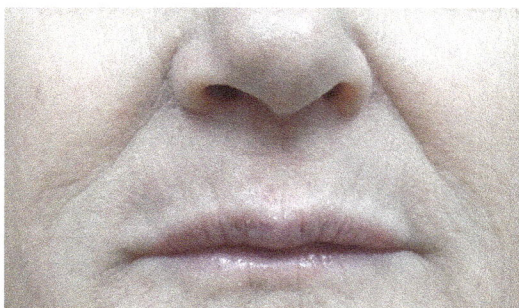

Revanesse® Versa™ Injection with TSK Microcannula

Pre-Revanesse® Versa™ in Nasolabial Fold

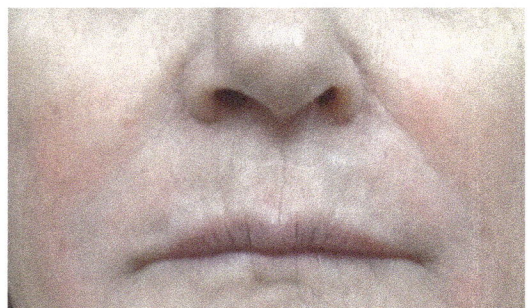

Post-Revanesse® Versa™ in Nasolabial Fold

39

Wiggle Progression Microcannula Technique

Traditionally, needles are blindly driven ahead regardless of obstruction, shearing tiny blood vessels which creates "the oozing which causes the bruising." Extravascular blood degrades and discolors over time to create unsightly ecchymosis, which can be more disconcerting to the patient than the treatment itself. Penetration of other soft tissues such as nerves, tendons, ligaments, and muscle invariably leads to swelling and pain. The microcannula advantage is that – with a little experience – the blunt tip makes it possible to almost touch sensitive tissue without actual penetration.

The "Wiggle Progression[33]" is simply to insert the microcannula through the Pilot hole and progress very slowly and gently – constantly prompting the patient to voice any significant pain – which is an indication of directly abutting the tissue we wish to bypass. With any report of pain, simply "Wiggle" back a bit and redirect the tip of the microcannula one or two millimeters in another direction or plane until no obstruction is felt, and then continue insertion until the desired end point is reached. We estimate a greater than 75% reduction in bruising using microcannula with the "Wiggle."

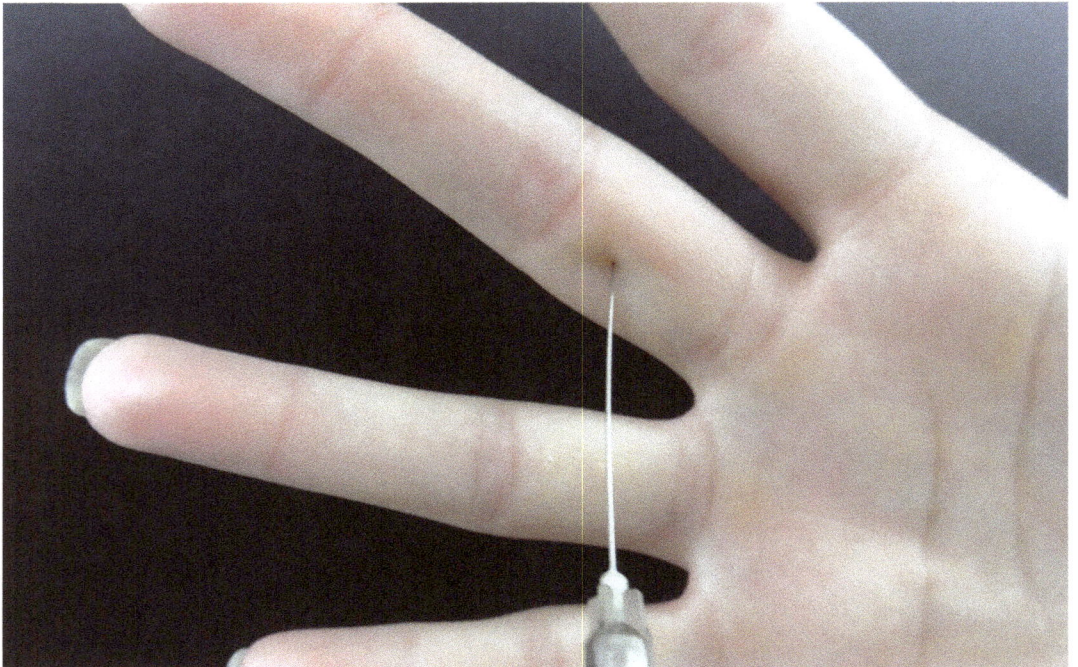

Microcannula Touching, Not Penetrating Obstruction (e.g. Blood Vessel)

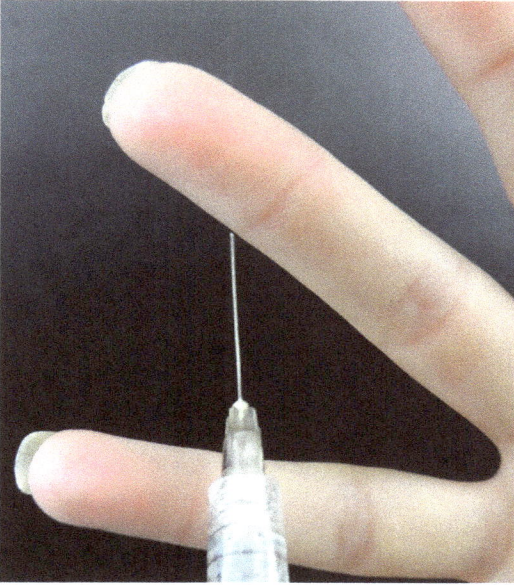
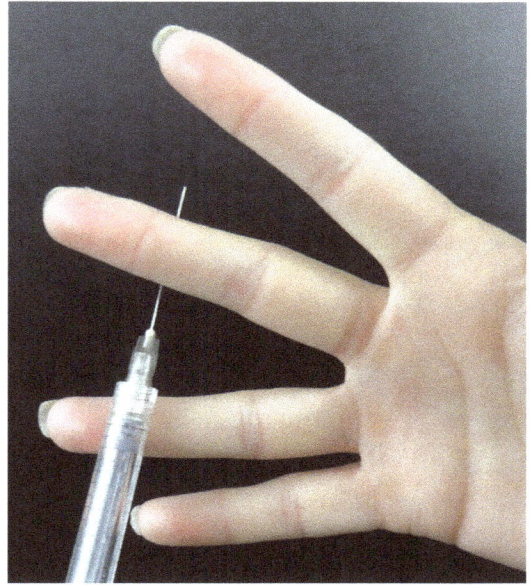

"Wiggle" Back, Move 1-mm in a Different Plane, Then Advanced Past the Obstruction

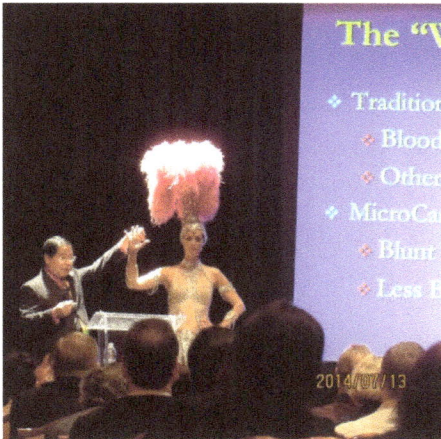
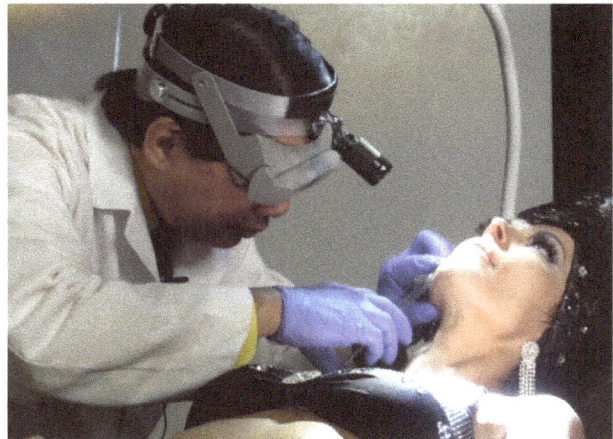

Dr. Lee Demonstrating the "Wiggle Progression" Upon Former Las Vegas Lead Showgirl

Submalar Technique
for Cosmetic Fillers

The submalar area,[39] just below the cheek, is an area in which many patients have also lost excessive fat volume. Care must be taken to only fulfill to the particular volume desire of each patient since a significant subset of patients will preferentially wish to maintain some volume loss here to give their face a more tapered appearance rather than that of complete fullness.

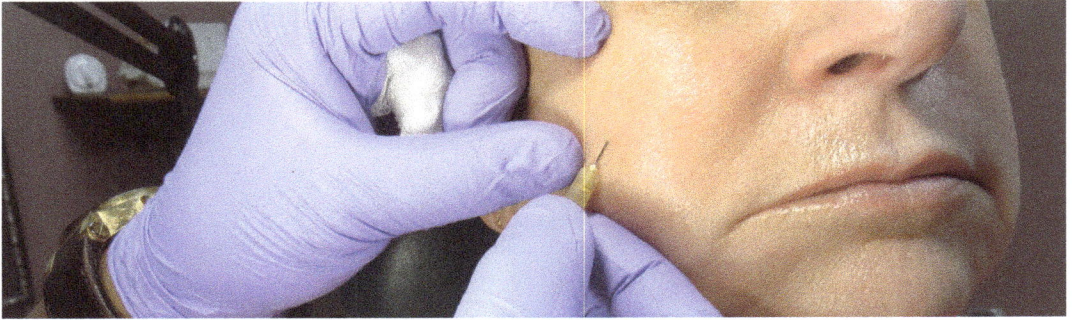

Pilot Needle and Microcannula Submalar Injection Using Basic Fan Technique

Again, the patient's desires supersede the physician's ideal sense of the aesthetic, so long as we maintain our conception of reasonable variations in the perception of normal cosmetically acceptable limits.

Our technique here is to overlay the microcannula tip over the area to be enhanced to plan out the entry point for the Pilot needle. Placement is dictated by setting the entry point to be able to have the microcannula reach the entirety or at least the majority of the desired area while it is ergonomically adjusted for the ease of the injector's placement.

We then simply enter and fan into the dermal-SQ junction after aspiration injecting retrograde and going forward with the Wiggle Progression Technique. Injection is in the superficial dermal-SQ junction to avoid penetration of the parotid gland and other important structures.

Upon completion, we repeat the process at a 90 degree angle to complete the Long MicroCannula Double Cross-Hatched Fan Technique (LeeXX).

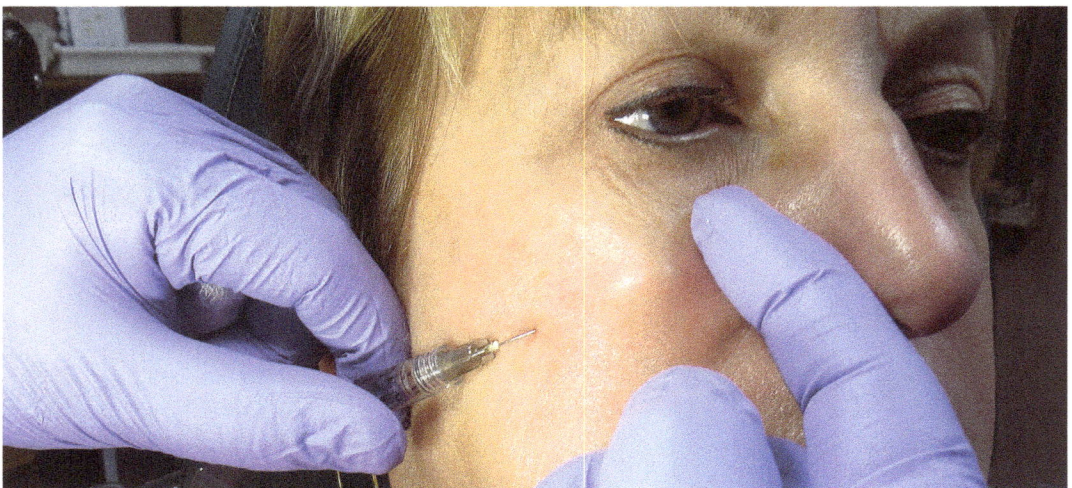

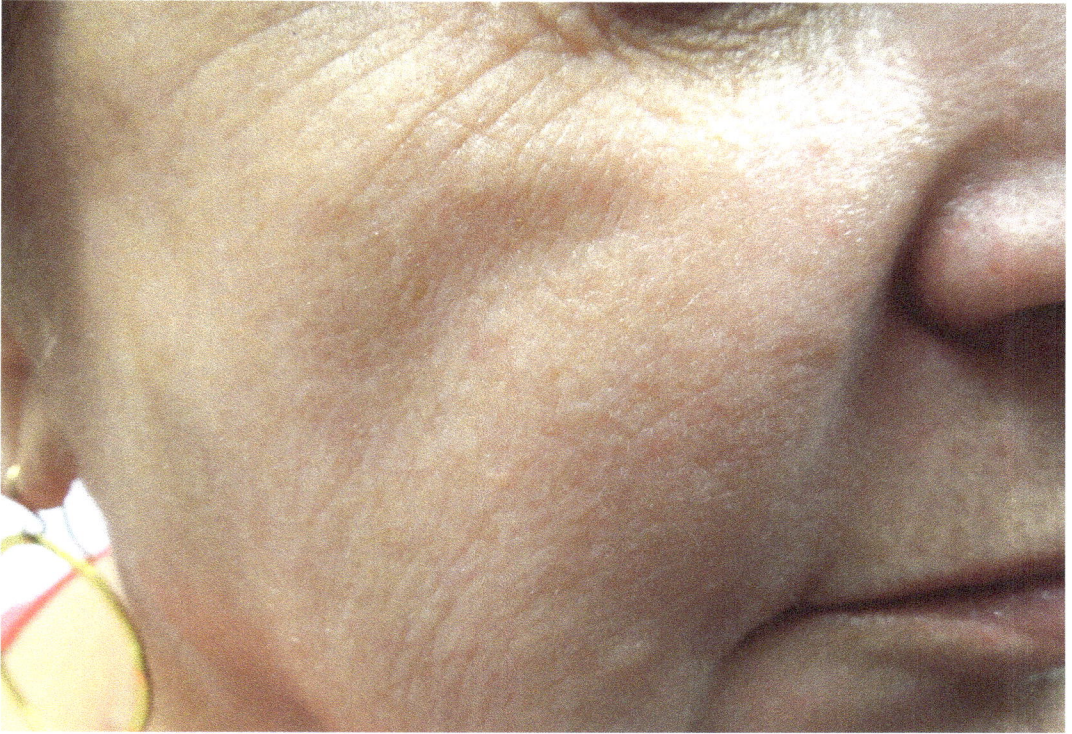

Pre/Post Treatment of Submalar With Juvederm Voluma® Injected by Microcannula

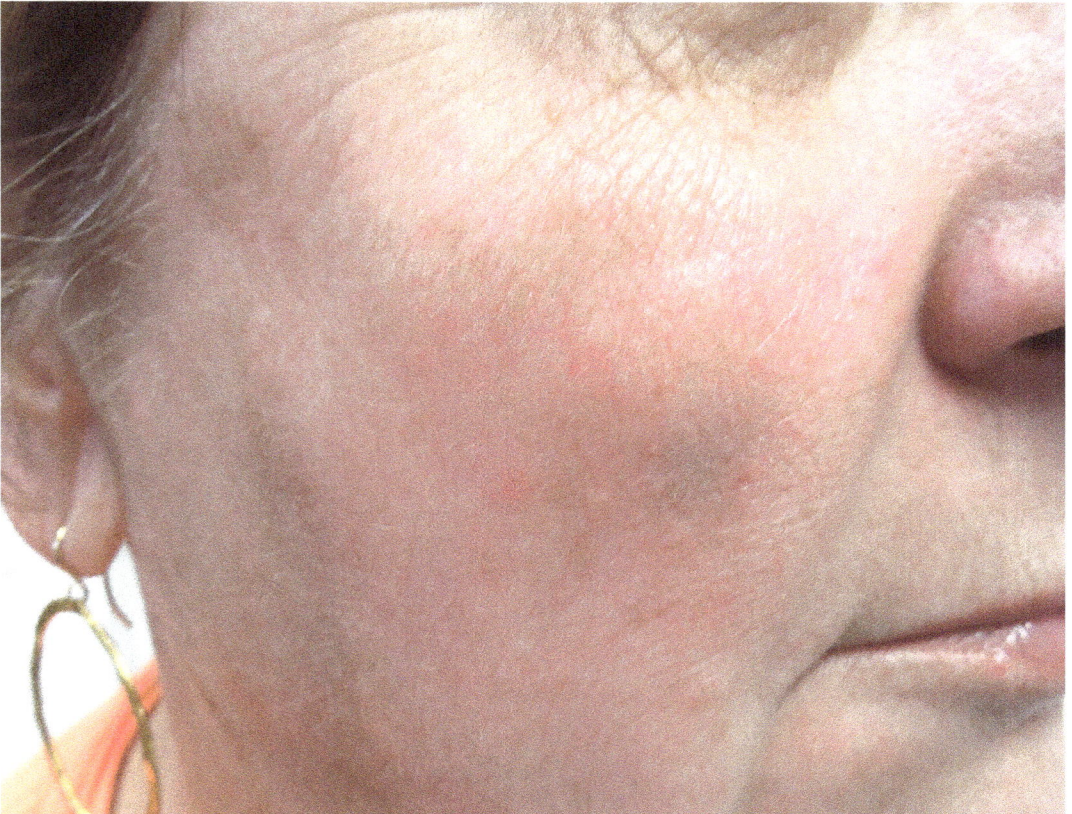

NOTES

Advanced Microcannula Facial Techniques

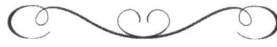

Lip Technique

Lips[40] are particularly difficult since even a minute variation in symmetry will often be examined most critically and with extreme close-up magnification by patients.

In the upper lip[41] we enter at the lateral aspect of the vermillion border, follow the vermillion border to Cupid's bow, then fan inferiorly into body of the upper lip as needed. In the lower lip, we enter at the lateral aspect of each side of the lip, insert to just past mid-line, then fan into the body of the lower lip as needed.

This is so atraumatic that I invariably use only topical numbing cream instead of the Inferior Orbital and Mental Nerve dental blocks which were so necessary using hypodermic needles.

Moreover, since there is so little trauma, it is far easier to create symmetric lips without swelling from multiple injections sites which can distort lip anatomy. One may also enhance Cupid's bow and the philtrum columns, but because only one injection is needed in each line, hypodermic needles with aspiration instead of microcannula should be used.

Additionally, we occasionally add other injection techniques to give a more voluptuous appearance to this baseline enhancement with microcannula. We also inject with a 27 gauge needle downwards from above the patient's head into the vermilion boarder in tiny aliquots aiming outwards which tends to pull the upper lip out into a more distinct pucker.

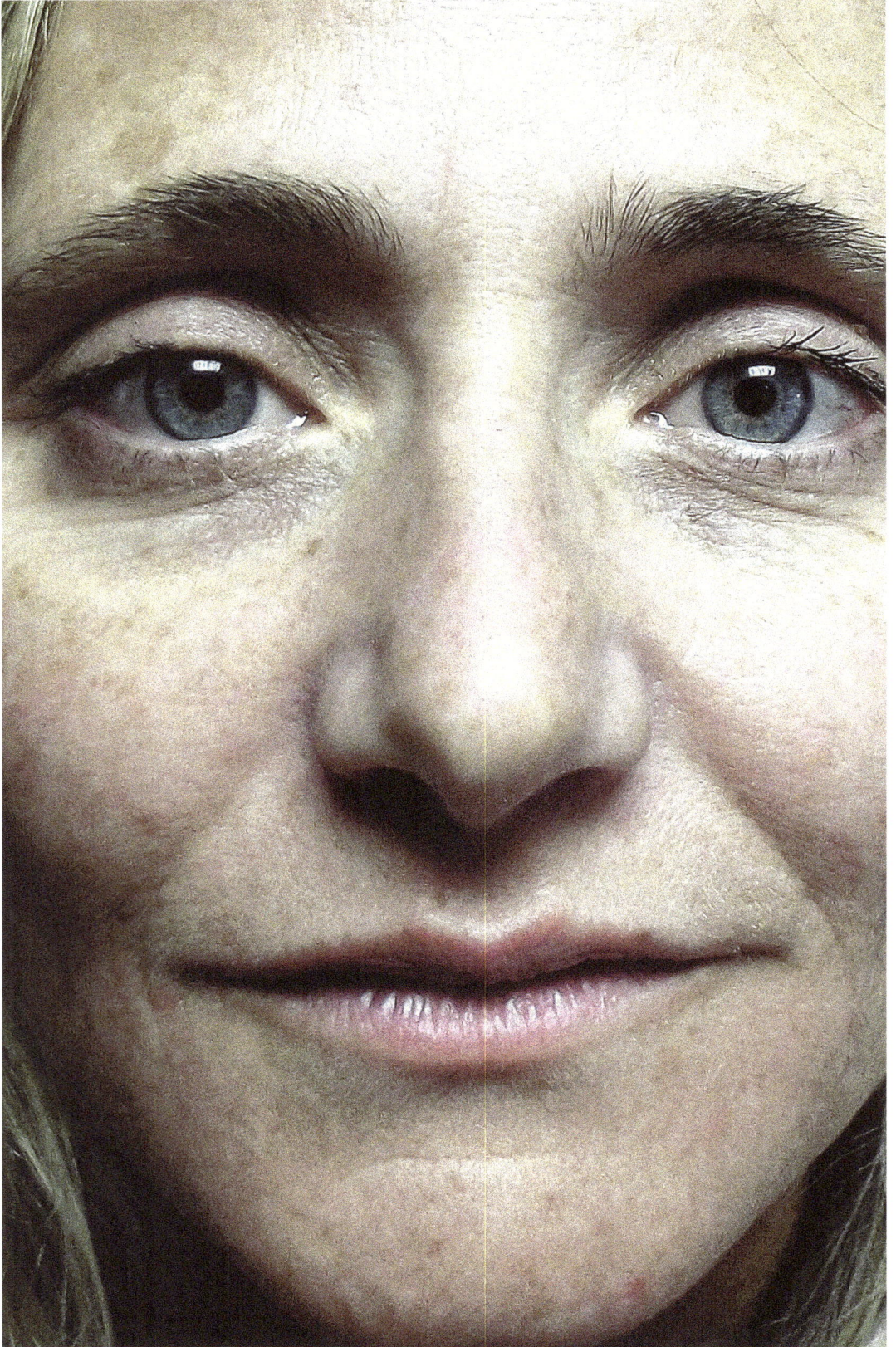

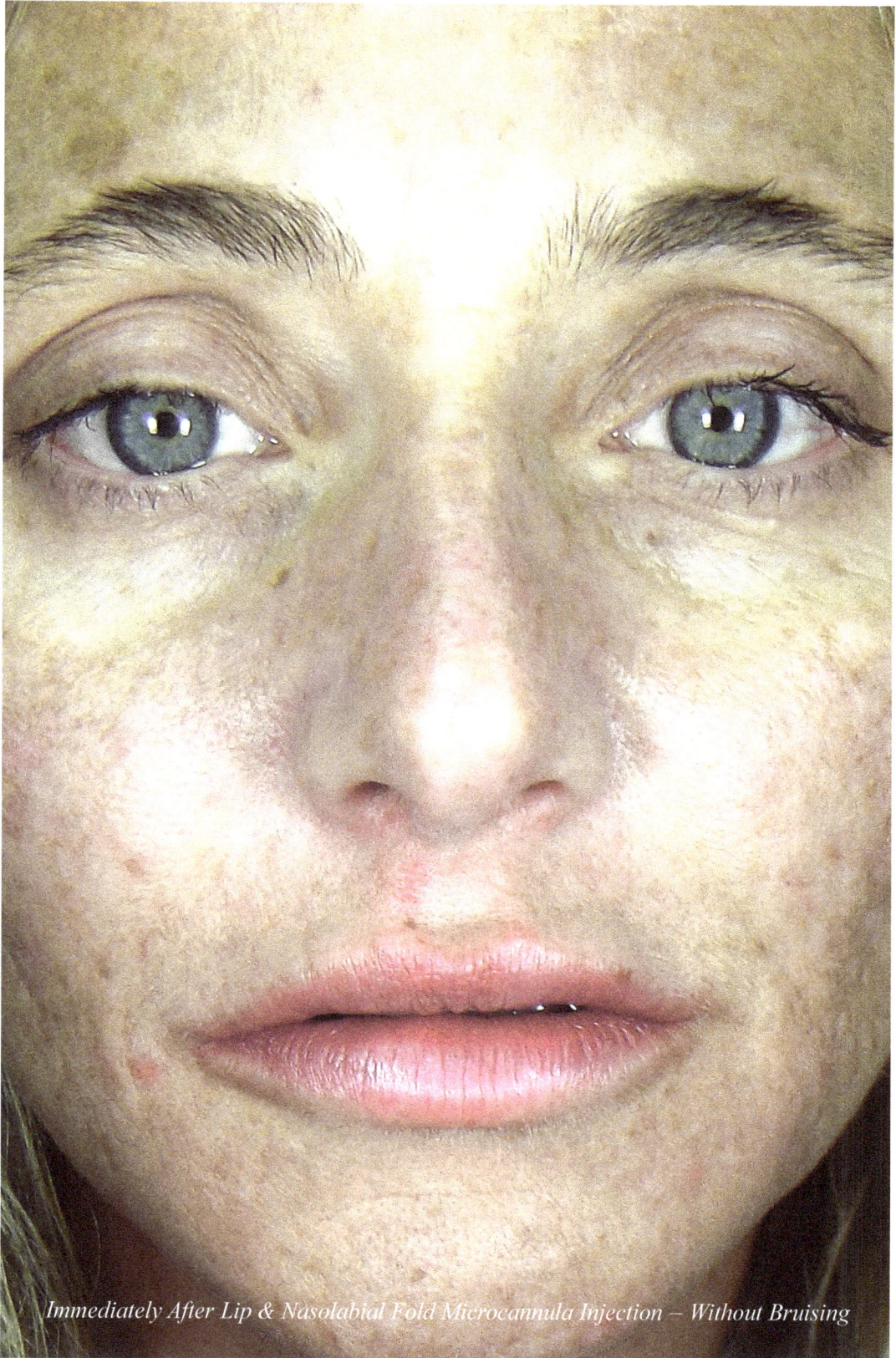

Immediately After Lip & Nasolabial Fold Microcannula Injection – Without Bruising

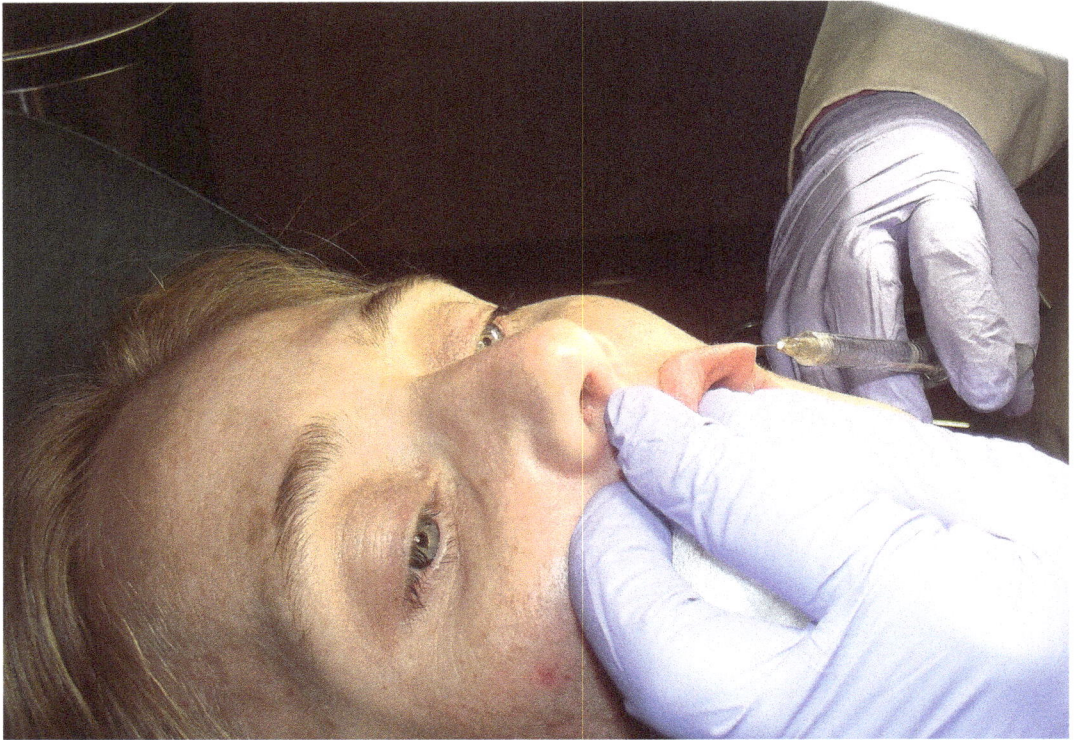

Juvederm Ultra Plus XC® Injection into Upper Lip with TSK STERiGLIDE Microcannula

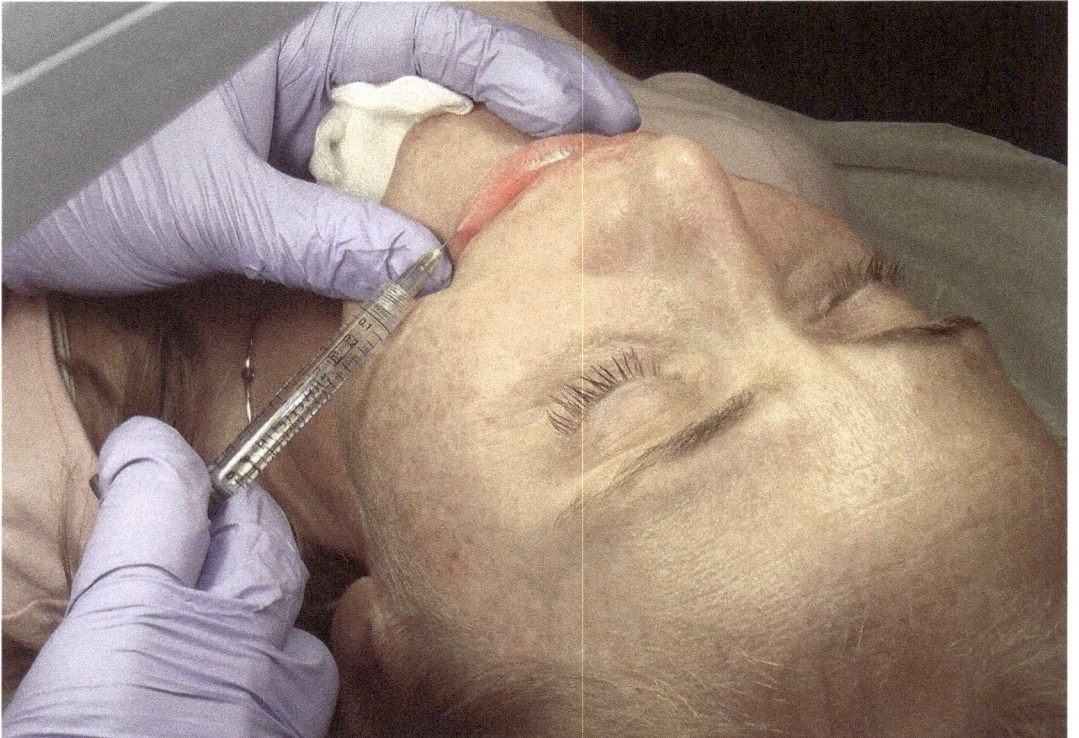

Lower Lip Technique with TSK STERiGLIDE Microcannula

MedEsthetics

BUSINESS EDUCAT[...] PRACTITIONERS

January/February 2017 $5.00
Volume 13, Number 1
medestheticsmagazine.com

Recognizing and Addressing
INJECTABLE
TREATMENT
COMPLICATIONS

PDT
FOR SKIN
REJUVENATION

Paul Vitenas Jr., MD
On His Custom-Built,
European-Inspired Aesthetic Care Center

Plus:
♦ Top Fillers for Lips
♦ Rosacea and Systemic Disease

BEFORE

AFTER

BEFORE

AFTER

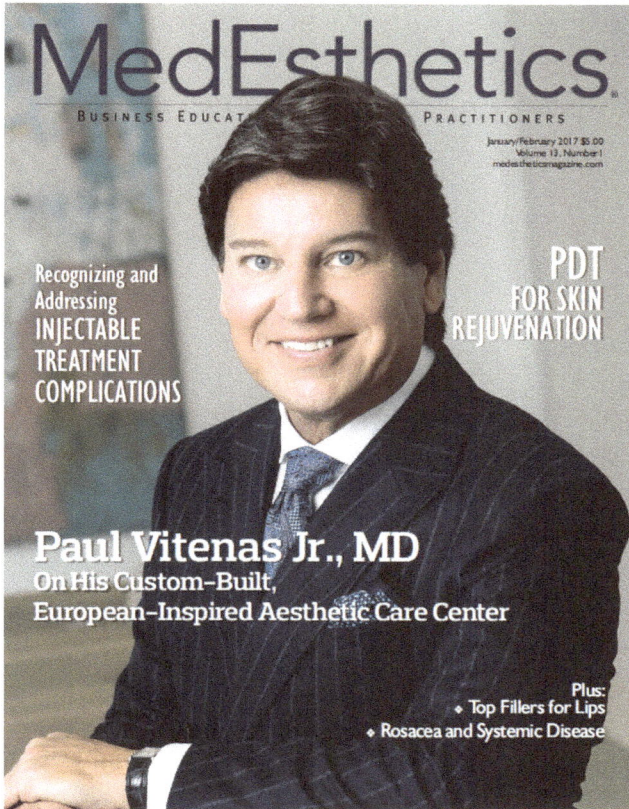

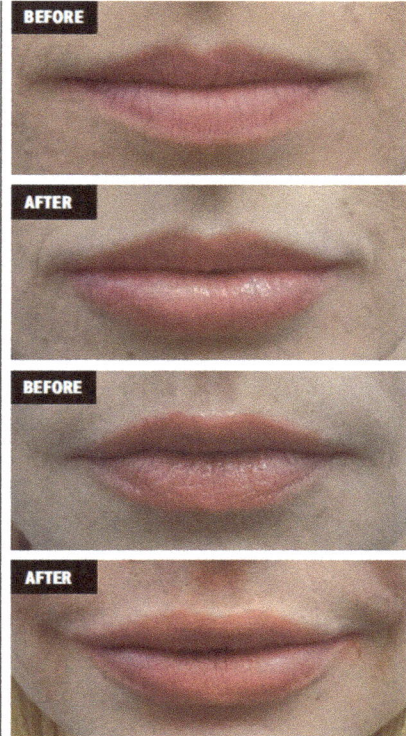

Dr. Garry R. Lee augmented the top patient's lips with Juvéderm Ultra and the bottom patient's using Juvéderm Volbella. He prefers the latter as it causes less postprocedure swelling.

The Lips of Dr. Lee's Patients Were Published Nationally as Ideal Lips in MedEsthetics

Cheek Technique

The greatest evolution in microcannula injection techniques is in the midface, which begins at the lower eyelid and ends at the oral commissure – and in particular – in how we inject to restore cheek volume.

Our approach in 2019 is to acknowledge that most midface volume loss is from the Deep Medial & Lateral Cheek Fat and the Suborbicularis Oculi Fat (SOOF), which acts like the structural foundation[28, 48] of the midface for the structures above. Separating these layers is the Superficial Muscular Aponeurotic System (SMAS), which functions much like a tissue wrapper separating compartments, but also allowing the passage of essential nerve and vascular conduits.

Consequently, when the deep foundation of cheek fat atrophies more rapidly as we age, the overlying superficial fat compartments – the infraorbital fat compartment, the medial and lateral superficial cheek compartment, and the nasolabial fat compartment – collapse into the chasm and sag in response to gravity in a downwards vector more from lack of structural foundation than from intrinsic superficial fat volume loss itself.

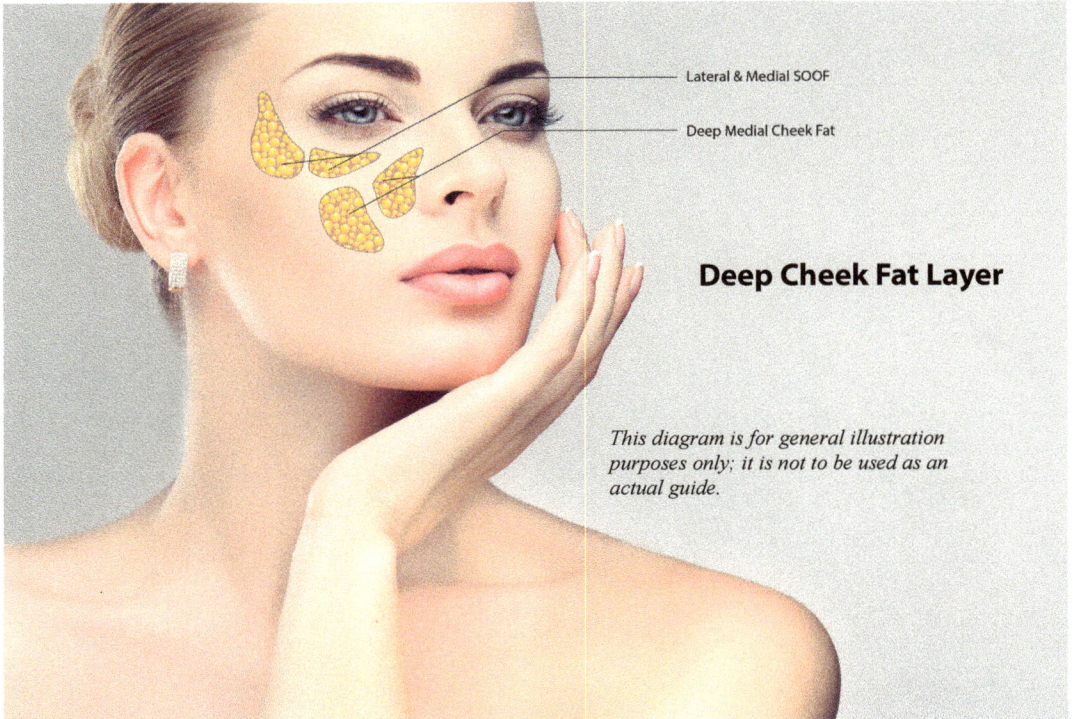

Lateral & Medial SOOF

Deep Medial Cheek Fat

Deep Cheek Fat Layer

This diagram is for general illustration purposes only; it is not to be used as an actual guide.

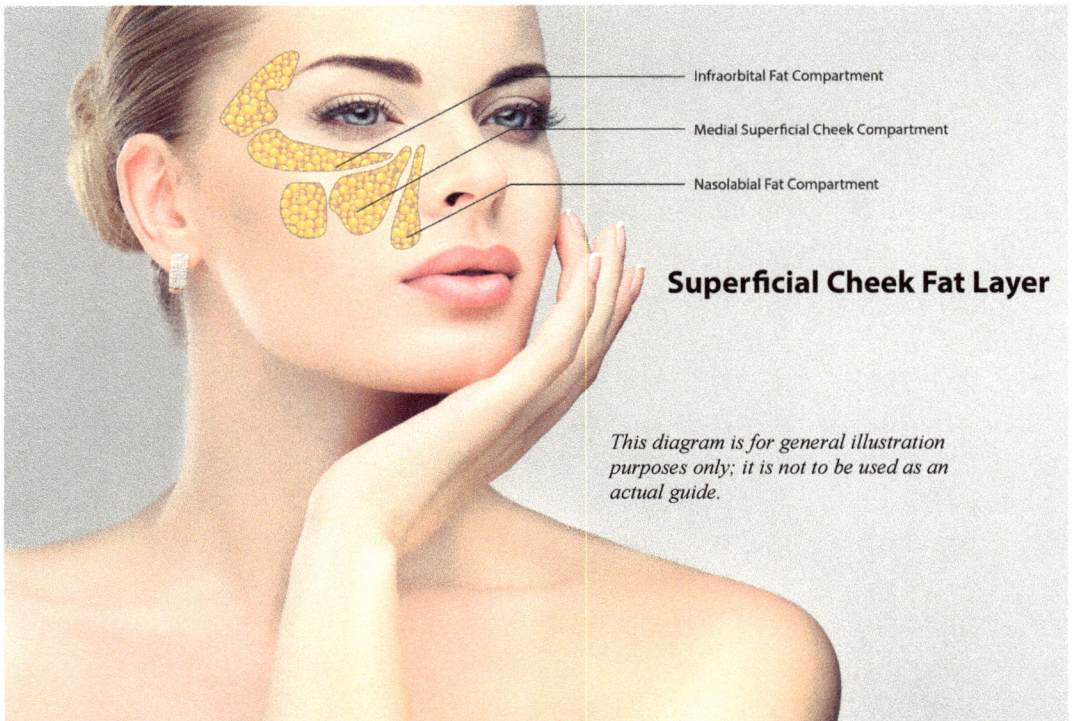

Infraorbital Fat Compartment

Medial Superficial Cheek Compartment

Nasolabial Fat Compartment

Superficial Cheek Fat Layer

This diagram is for general illustration purposes only; it is not to be used as an actual guide.

Of course, contributing factors to aging besides fat volume loss also include bony resorption, skin thinning, increased skin laxity, and muscle atrophy.

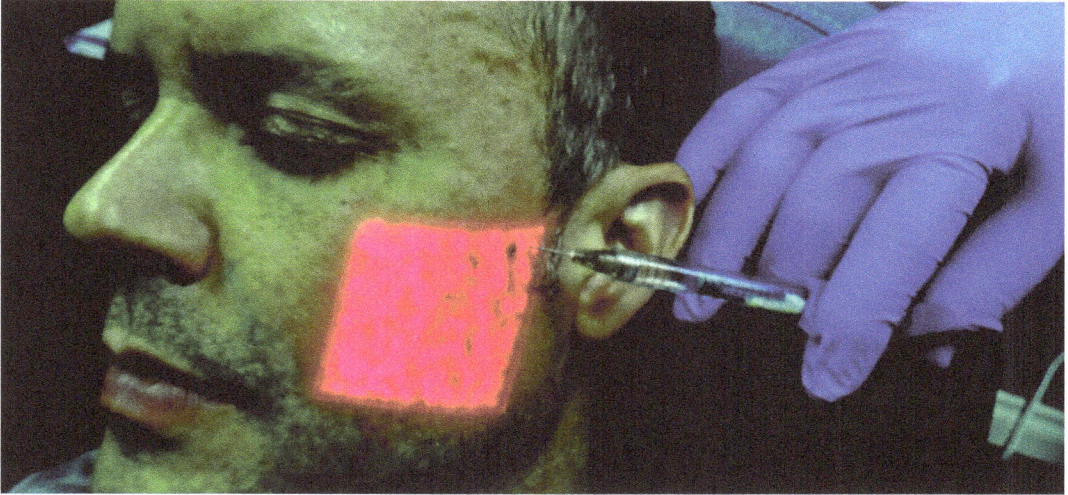

First, I use the AccuVein™ [29] laser imaging system to illuminate the in vivo location of each patient's actual blood vessels in the area I plan to inject, with a precision – according to AccuVein™ – of up to 1.0 cm deep and the width of a strand of hair. The AccuVein,™ however, will not detect arteries deeper than 1.0 cm with thicker vessel walls and since the AccuVein™ light may obscure the shadowing of skin – which I use in real time to estimate the need for more depth correction – I now just have one of our assistants draw in the major blood vessels in the area of concern with a skin marking pencil. When drawn in – or mapped – my own hands don't interfere with the laser light illumination of our patient's blood vessels when I inject cosmetic filler.

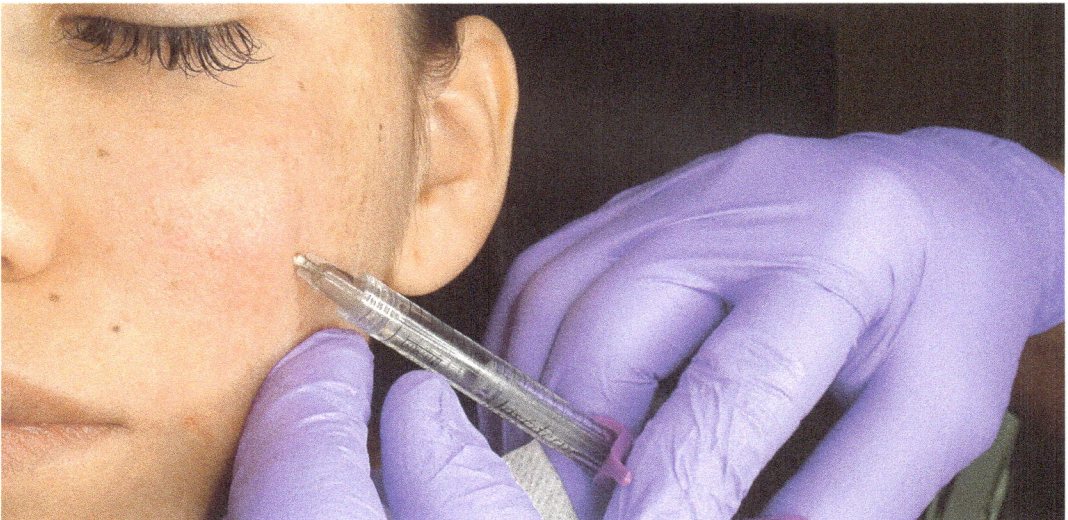

Second, for the cheek, I insert the Pilot needle lateral to the mid-pupillary line approximately where it intersects a horizontal line from the ala of the nose in the direction of the deep medial cheek fat, just below the Tear Trough, a minimally vascular zone. Instead of the usual superficial Pilot needle minimal injection depth into the dermal-SQ junction, we now aim the Pilot deep and directly at the Deep Medial Cheek Fat.

Keep in mind our placement is only an estimate of each patient's actual anatomy, since standard diagrams cannot precisely place vasculature due to anatomic variations, much less realignment after surgery or trauma. Moreover, the absence of AccuVein™ markings is not proof that deeper undetected arteries do not lie below or that our assistant has marked every visible vessel.

I then insert the microcannula deep in the direction of the Deep Medial Cheek Fat tunneling to just above the periosteum using the Wiggle Progression Technique, then fan into the Deep Lateral Cheek Fat.

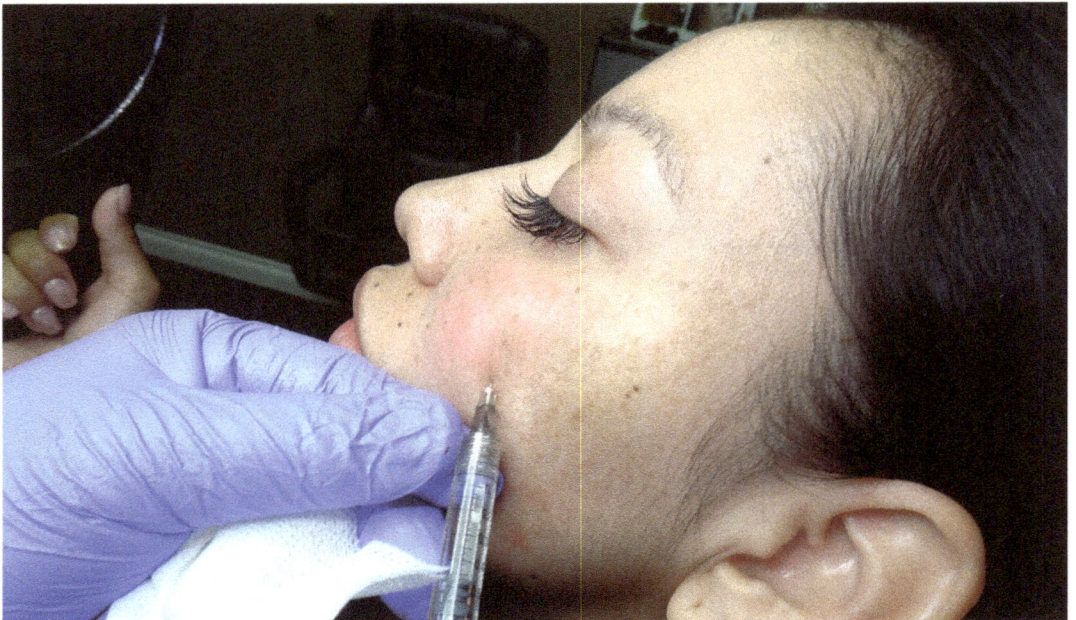

At times, you can actually feel the microcannula tip gently "pop" into this space, validating your positioning. I slowly and gently bolus the filler in retrograde until it re-inflates the fat pad to give me the visual appearance I want – just below the Tear Trough to ~90% correction – to allow for subsequent swelling.

I then fan the microcannula medially and laterally to re-create a deep supporting structure with particular care to avoid the angular artery and vein and the facial artery and tributaries using the Wiggle Progression Technique.

Often, this alone is satisfactory to the patient; however I also fan to the sub-orbicularis oculi fat (SOOF) with the same process to inflate it to the visual aspect I desire just above the periosteum. Care must be taken to not over-do the lateral SOOF which may potentially interfere with lymphatic drainage in this area.

Again, the current thought is that the deep fat compartments preferentially deflate with aging and the superficial fat compartments are relatively preserved creating a drooping effect over the lower face. Hence, re-inflation essentially re-builds the structural support below the superficial fat layers re-creating the original youthful appearance.

However, if the Tear Trough deficit is profound, re-building only the foundation may actually result in accentuating the depth of the Tear Trough. Our solution is then to inject minute amounts of Belotero Balance® just above the periosteum with microcannula with at least 50% undercorrection, due to expected swelling (see Tear Trough Section).

Typically, this re-inflation also provides structural support for the orbital retaining ligament and significantly improves the Tear Trough area, perhaps to the point that no additional treatment is needed in the Tear Trough. It also lifts the midface back to where it was, often greatly reducing the depth of the nasolabial fold, the marionette lines, and the jowl over the mandible.

Also note that when I use the word "lift," it is not truly a lift because we are limited by cosmetic filler injection to only increasing the face's forward projection. True lift can only be accomplished with surgery or threadlift, though energy type devices can also tighten skin to produce a modest lift.

Our preferred HA cheek fillers in the deep and superficial fat compartments are Juvederm Voluma® or Restylane Lyft® for their higher G' properties, their elastic behavior when deformed defined in rheology as the Stress/Strain.

We prefer to sequence cosmetic filler injections from the cheek first, then follow by injecting the nasolabial fold because the lateral-superior placement in the cheek often markedly reduces the severity of the nasolabial folds by anchoring the skin so less product is needed medially.

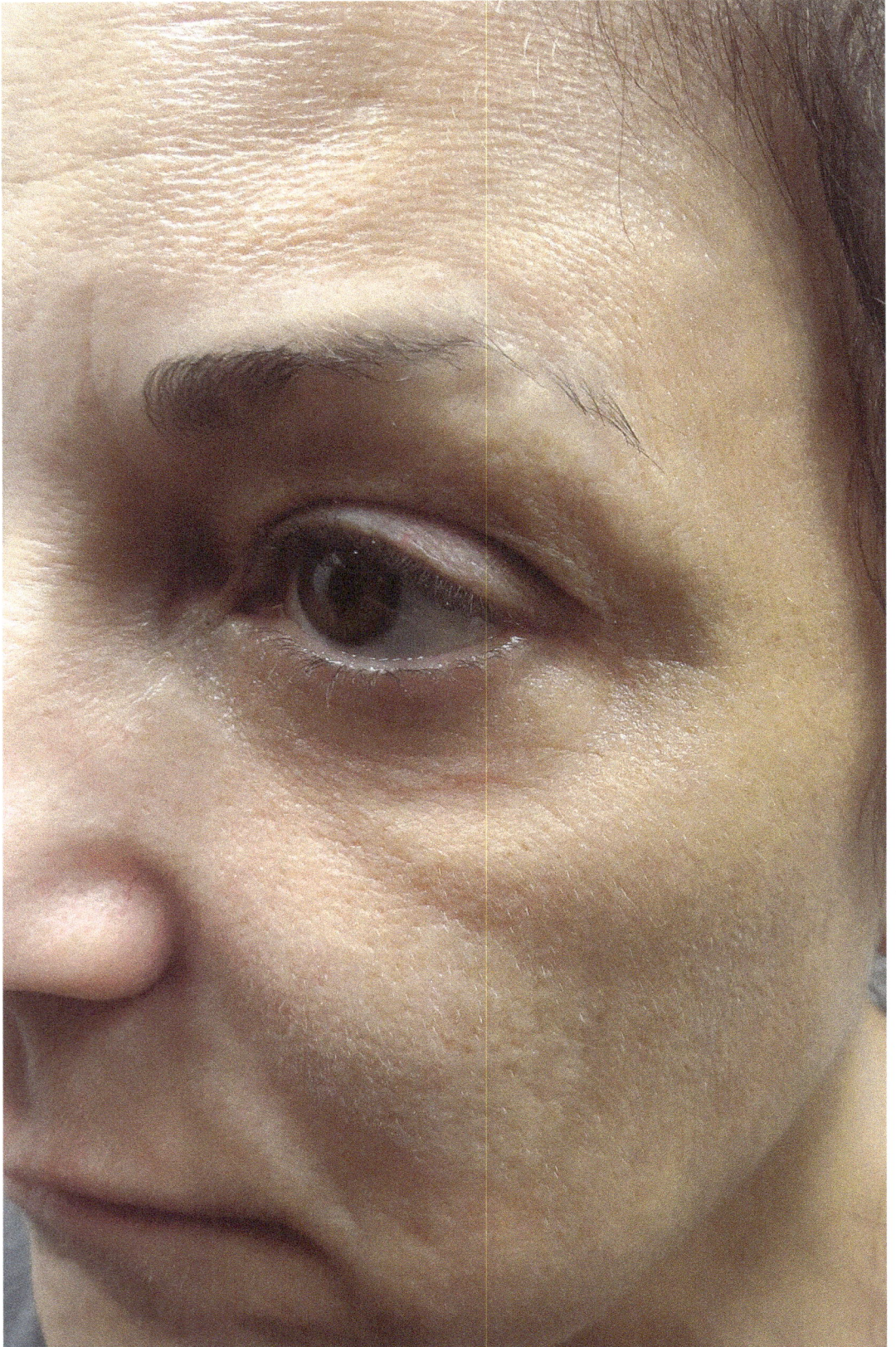

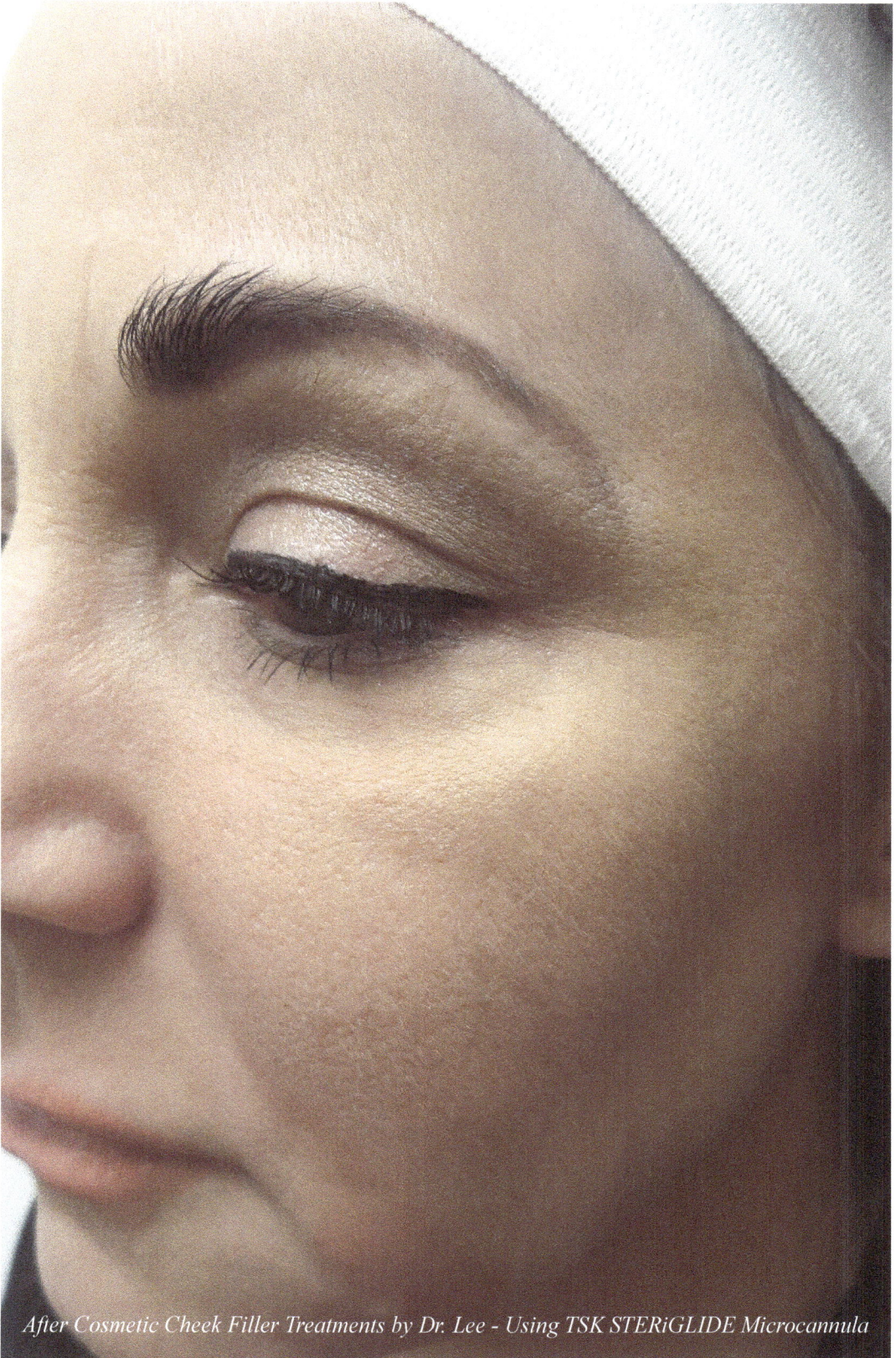

After Cosmetic Cheek Filler Treatments by Dr. Lee - Using TSK STERiGLIDE Microcannula

I use a process I call "traction estimation" to more precisely place injection sites in the cheek and submalar areas by applying traction upwards to simulate amount of lift with a given volume of filler and to identify the key tension points which cause the most significant lift.

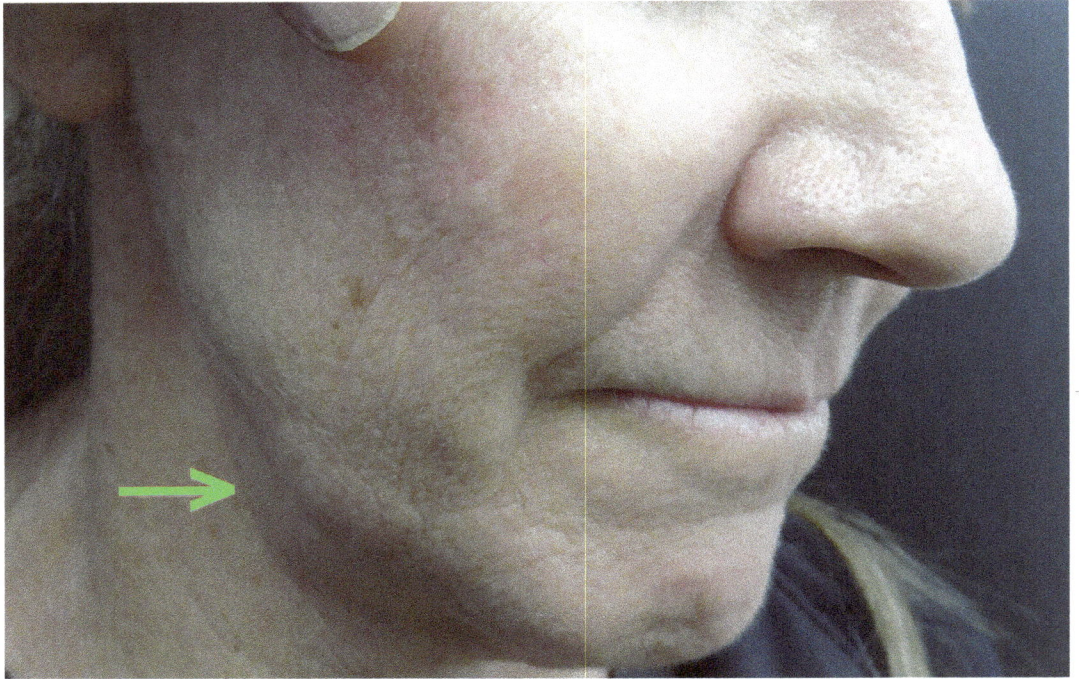

"Traction Estimation" to Determine the Effect of Placement of Cosmetic Fillers in Cheek

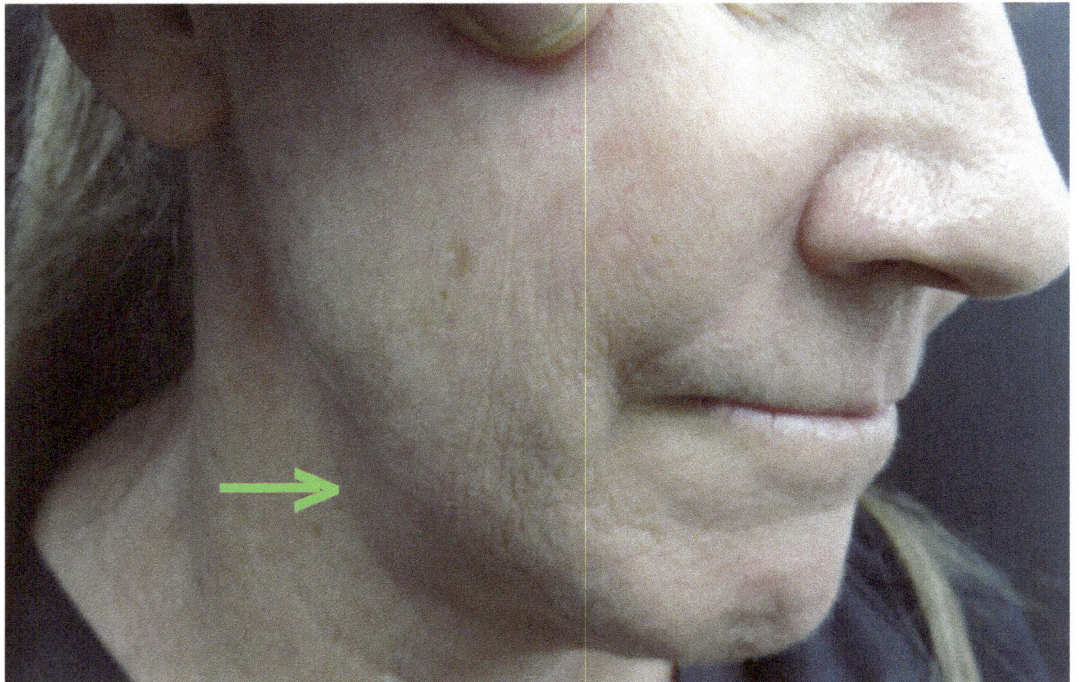

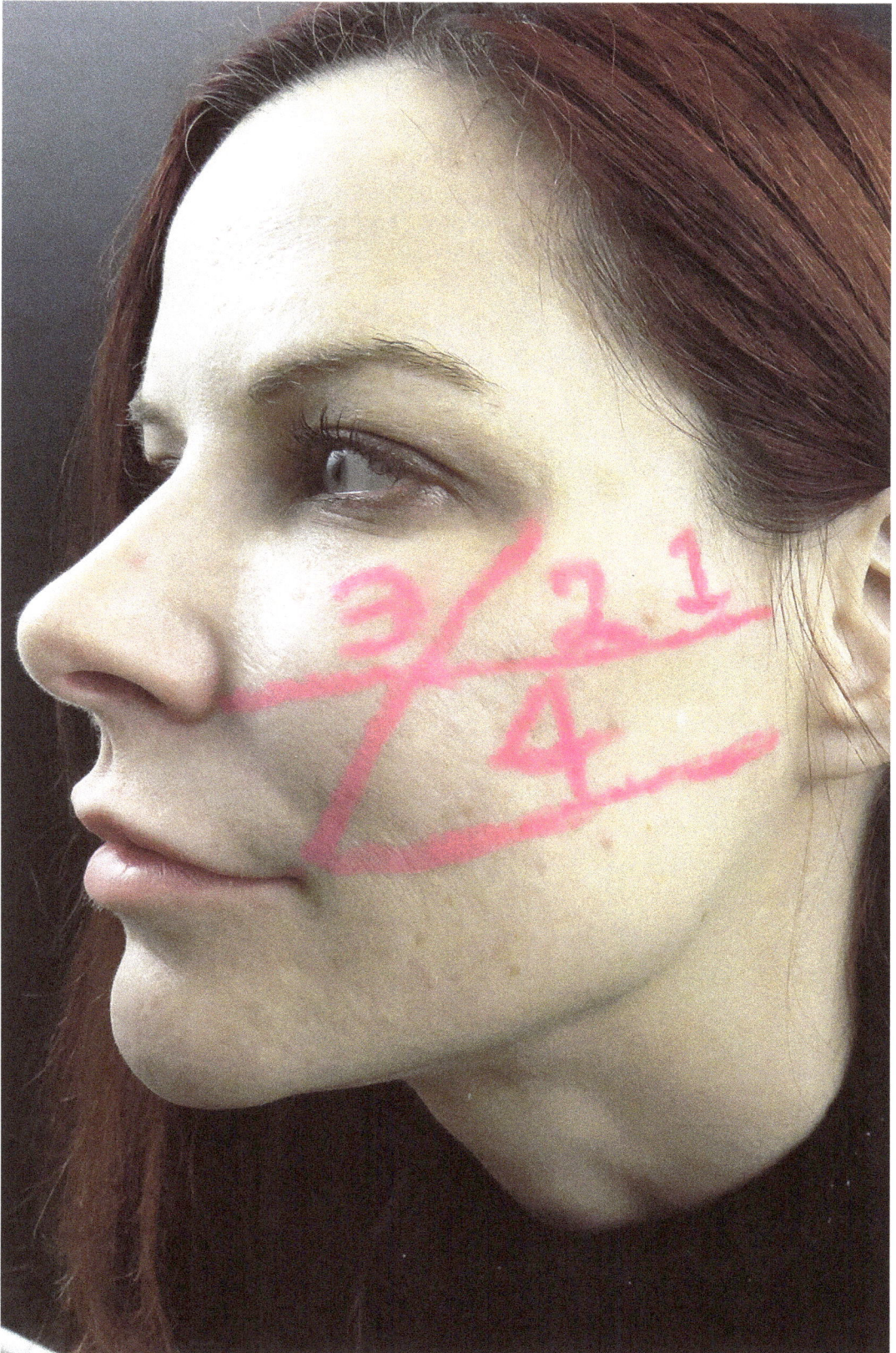

Traditional Hypodermic Needle Technique

In contrast to my injection technique cited above, the On-Label conventional method of injecting Juvederm Voluma® is to demarcate Hinderer's Lines,[39] the two lines that the cross midface highlighting the malar prominence of the cheek. Hinderer's lines divide the cheek into four distinct zones which should be injected sequentially in order to give the most efficient lift to the cheek. Line #1 is from the lateral canthus to the oral commissure and line #2 is from the tragus of ear to upper alar lobule of the nose.

These result in the classic four (4) injection sites: the Zygomatic Arch at sites 1-2 which anchor and lift laterally; the Anteromedial Zone at site 3; and finally the Submalar Zone at site 4. Injections are then made using needles perpendicular to the skin placed supra-periosteal in sites 1-2; and above the periosteum, but into the subcutaneous tissue in the remaining sites.

Tear Trough Technique

The Tear Trough is the depression of the medial lower eyelid just lateral to the anterior lacrimal crest, limited inferiorly by the inferior orbital rim.[42] This is an area only for advanced injectors because of the higher risk of retinal artery cannulation, which may result in permanent blindness.[34, 43, 44] Other risks include stroke and necrosis leading to ulcer formation and scarring. Microcannula use is deemed safer because the blunt tip is thought to be less likely to penetrate blood vessels, but of course, if enough force is applied, penetration can also occur with microcannula.

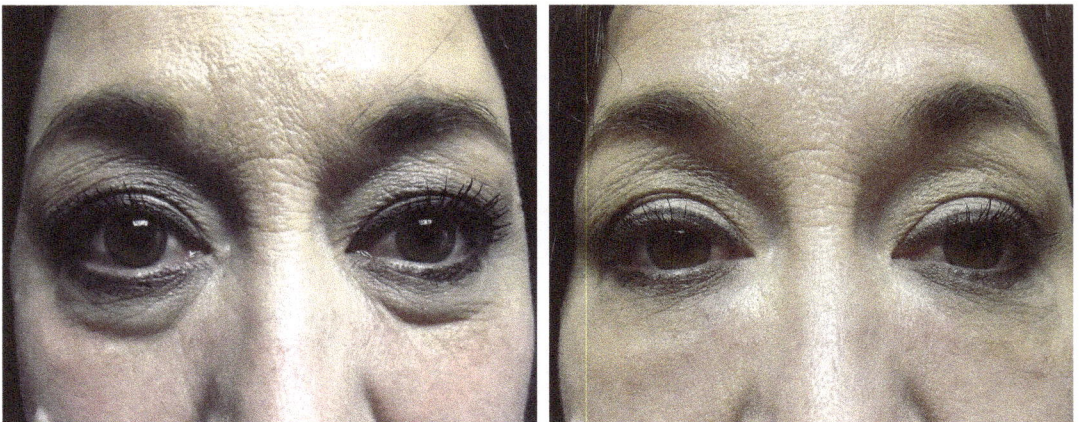

Before and After Cosmetic Filler Injections with TSK STERiGLIDE Microcannula

Another peculiar observation I made in this area is the tendency for hyperpigmentation[45, 46] to be naturally present here which may create the appearance of volume loss even when corrected. Consequently, our protocol is to take high resolution digital photography and to point out the difference between volume loss and the shadowing effect versus skin discoloration – prior to Tear Trough treatment. Indeed, hyperpigmentation becomes even more evident when no longer hidden by involution in loose skin folds after cosmetic filler volume correction. The other salient issue I observed is the occasional tendency of the hyaluronic acid fillers I have used to spontaneously swell days, weeks, or months after the initial swelling has subsided, requiring enzymatic correction. Our experience is that Belotero Balance® is the least likely of the HA cosmetic injectable fillers to swell, but nevertheless, we still note significant swelling so our current protocol is to under-treat this area with just minute amounts of Belotero® injected just above the periosteum with extreme care with microcannula using the Wiggle Progression Technique.

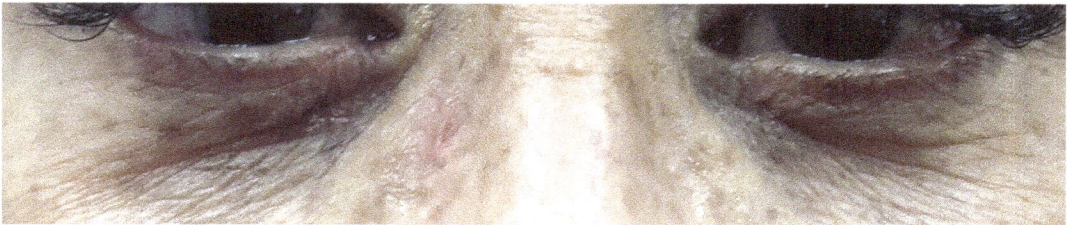

Skin Hyperpigmentation Hidden in Tear Trough
Shadow Becomes More Visible After Volume Replacement

My Tear Trough approach in 2019 is to first treat the cheek deformity because for many patients, re-volumizing the Deep Medial Cheek Fat is sufficient to also tighten the skin laxity above in the Tear Trough, which is just superior and medial to the inferior orbital rim. My preferred cheek filler in 2019 is Restylane Lyft® or Juvederm Voluma,® inserted deep primarily for their G' capacity to build a foundation for the mid-face. If the improvement injecting the Deep Medial Cheek Fat below is insufficient in tightening the Tear Trough above, we use Belotero Balance® in the skin above because Juvederm Voluma® and Restylane Lyft® are too thick – with a tendency for lumpiness – for superficial placement in the thin eyelid skin just above the orbital rim.

In our first book, we used Restylane Silk® in the Tear Trough area, but in 2019, we prefer Belotero Balance® to tighten loose skin with minimal swelling when placed deep below the dermal-SQ junction. Our concept is that the Deep Medial Cheek Fat forms the foundation of the midface structure and correction has to begin at the foundation first to recreate the anatomical appearance of youth without distortion. Correction of the Tear Trough first – independent of the foundation – may actually enhance apparent prolapse of the superficial structures, particularly with respect to the proximate restraining ligaments. Again, with Belotero Balance,® under-correction is recommended, as every HA filler will be hydrophilic to some degree and under correction is always preferable aesthetically to over correction. Currently, we recommend at least a 30% under correction, to be re-evaluated a week or two later for refinement, if necessary. Note that the more volume deficiency is corrected, the more likely the patient is to notice swelling, as the skin become increasingly level with the surrounding area. Swelling in a volume depleted area, or skin depression, is less visibly apparent or may even be perceived as improvement by the patient. Consequently, the closer the patient is to full correction, the more likely the patient is to swell excessively.

Tear Trough Technique

Our Tear Trough technique is to first map the larger blood vessels in the area with the AccuVein™ laser device, which illuminates blood vessels up to 1.0 centimeters in depth, using a surgical marker. This minimizes the chances of accidentally inserting injectable filler into a blood vessel by avoiding the areas indicated by the surgical marker. My preferred entry point is lateral to the ala of the nose, just lateral to the horizontal intersection with the vertical mid-pupillary line, a relatively avascular area. We then inject just above the periostium after aspiration, intentionally under-treating the area to avoid swelling.

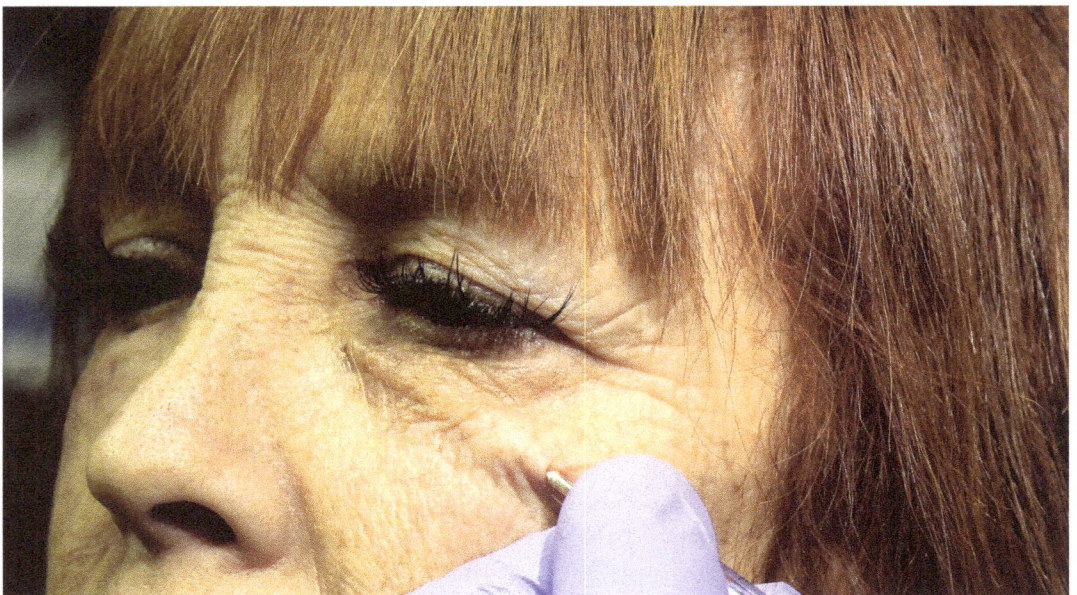

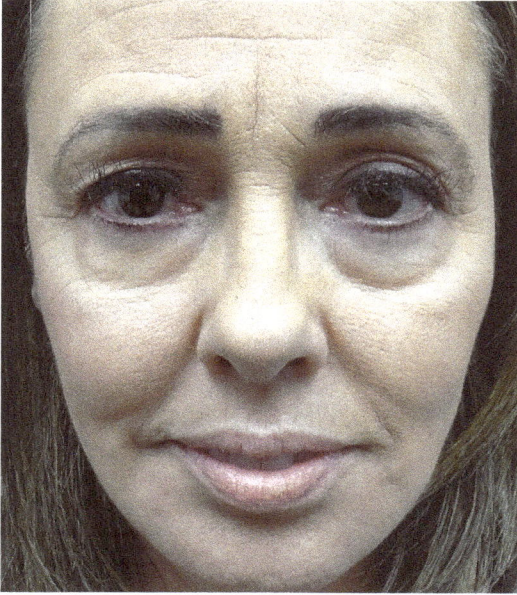

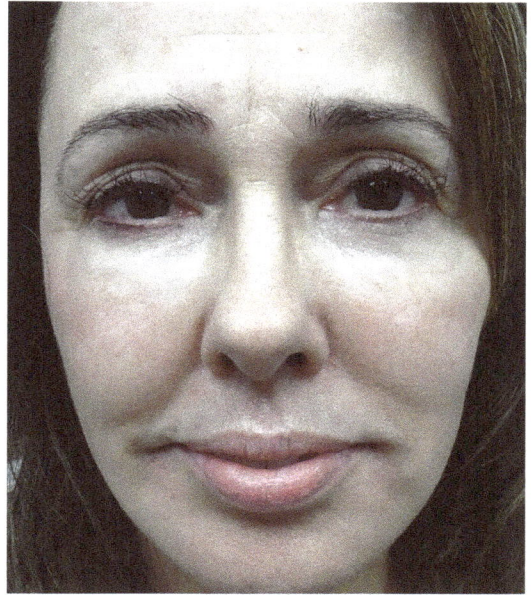

Racoon Eye Volume Deformity Corrected by Dr. Lee with Belotero® and Restylane Lyft®

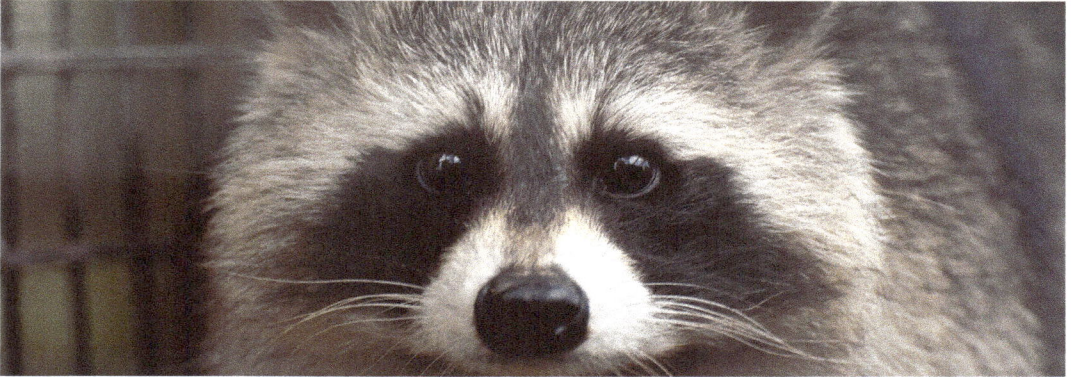

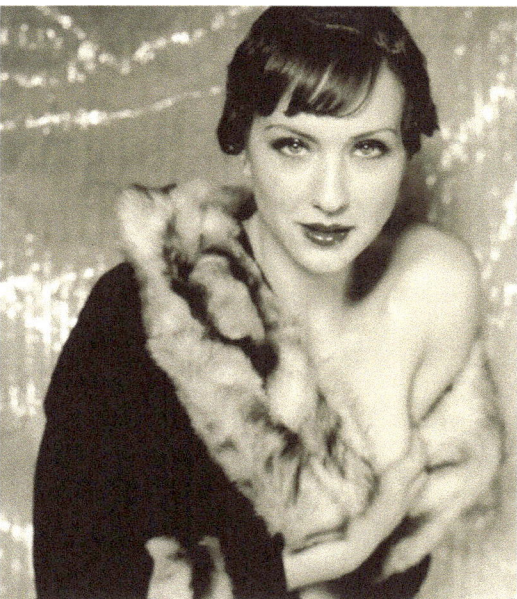

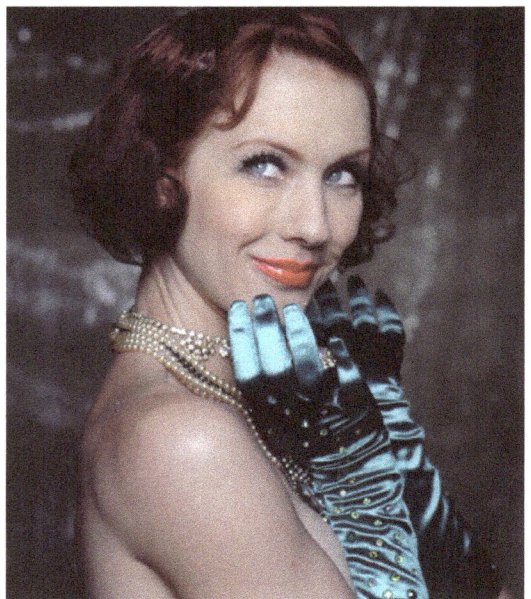

With Belotero Balance,® we no longer pre-treat with Prednisone to minimize post-treatment swelling because there is usually minimal swelling with deep enough placement and adequate under correction. However, Medrol DosePak can easily be added after treatment, if necessary.

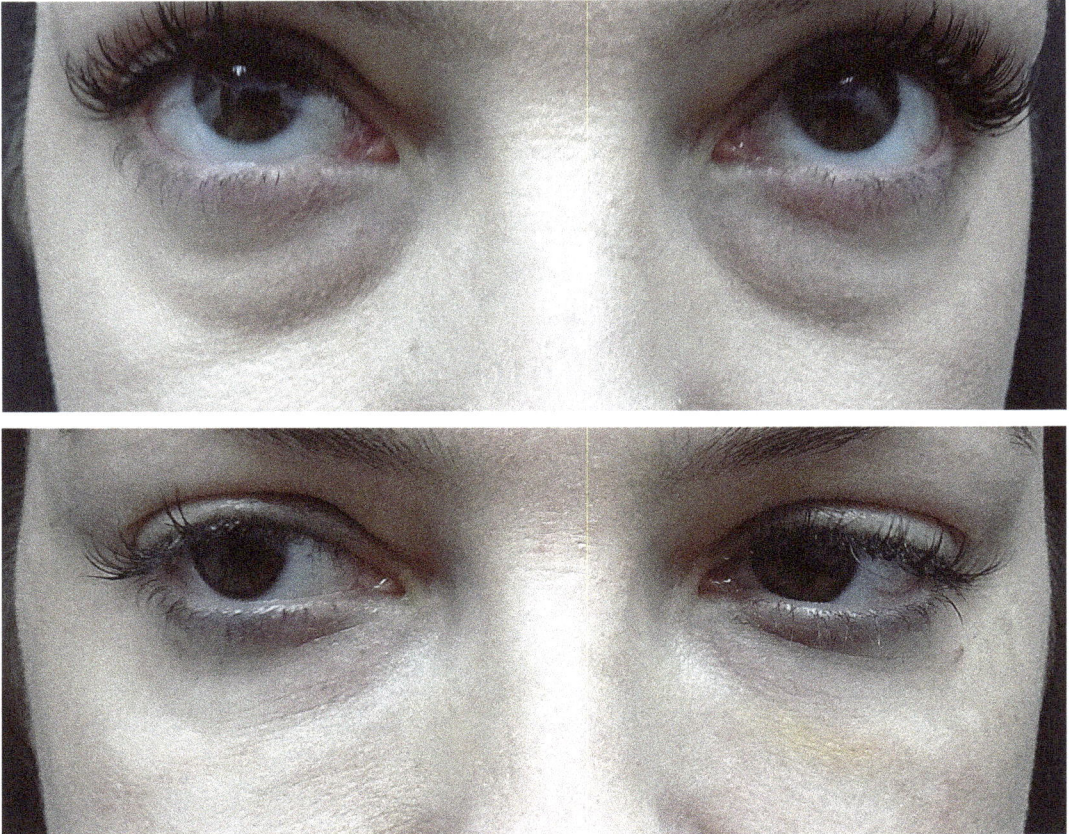

Fifty Percent (50%) Correction of Tear Trough Using TSK STERiGLIDE Microcannula

Overcorrection will occasionally require the use of Hylenex,[47] the recombinent form of the enzyme Hyaluronidase, which we use judiciously at least a week or two after the last injection to make sure we are not attempting to dissolve apparent excessive product – which is actually unresolved swelling. We use Hylenex Off-Label because it does not require skin allergy testing as it is not formulated with animal derived proteins.

Of all the cosmetic injection areas we treat, the Tear Trough is the most difficult to meet patient expectations and the most likely to require correction or to have complications, so it should be reserved for only the most experienced preceptorship trained clinicians for patients who are not obsessed with expectations of perfection.

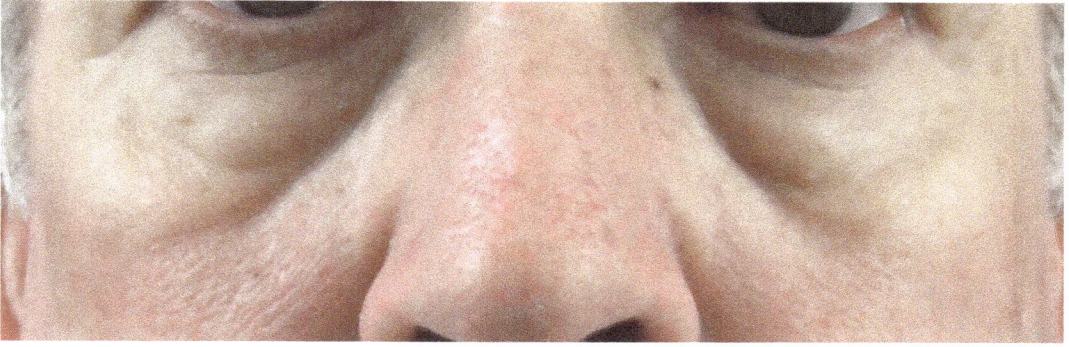

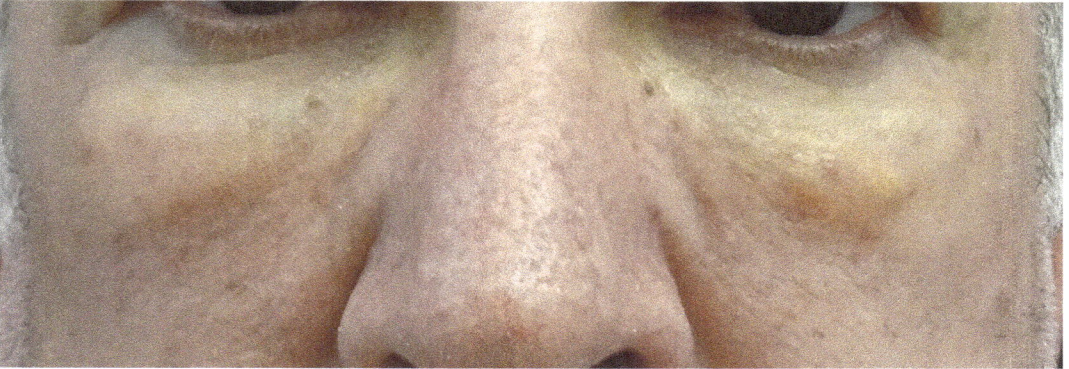

Correction of Tear Trough Using TSK STERiGLIDE Microcannula

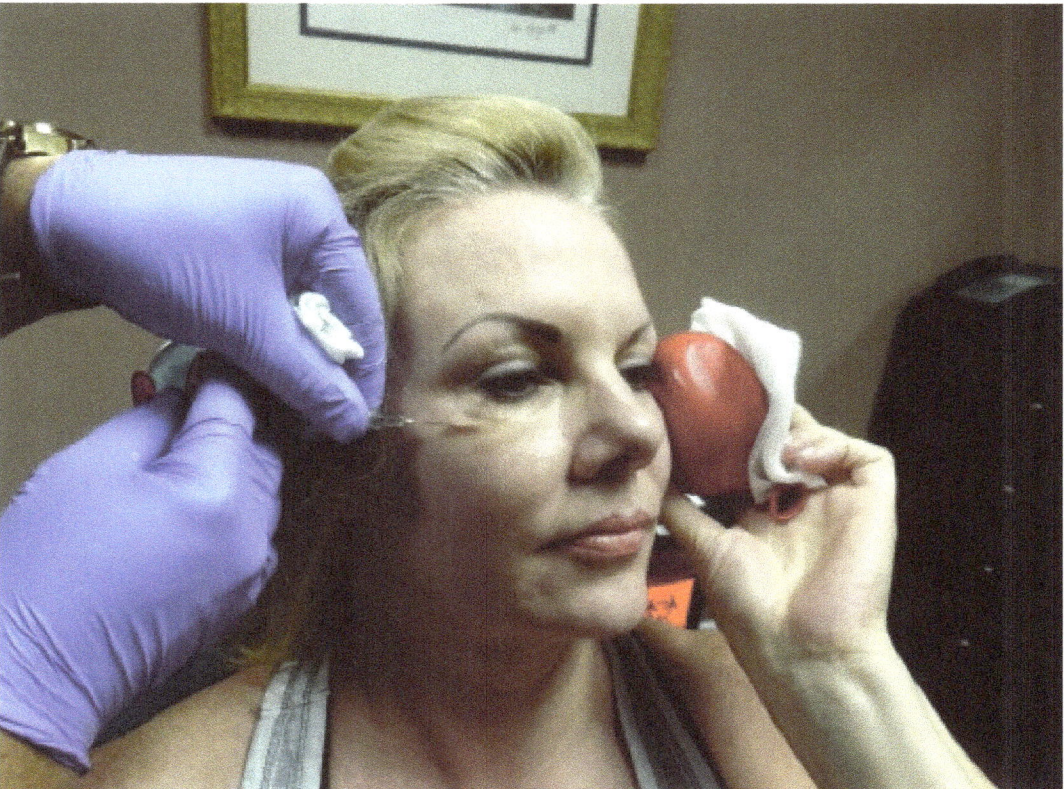

Pre-Auricular Technique
for Cosmetic Fillers

The Pre-Auricular area of the midface is simply the area in front of the ear. Aesthetically, it can transition into the Submalar area and form a continuum or become a separate but distinct area of volume loss apart from the Submalar area with aging. Its importance is that loss of volume here causes subsequent issues of the aesthetic in areas below it and medial and lateral to it, since skin laxity here contributes to an increase in the jowl area around the mandible as well as the marionette area at the lower aspect of the mouth. When present in youth, it provides support to the adjacent anatomic structures below it, just as its diminution invariably undermines the support of dependent facial anatomical structures below.

I treat the pre-auricular area particularly when I want to increase skin traction towards a diagonal or lateral vector from the skin and tissue around the mouth towards the ear. This gives the appearance of a diagonal lift, though it is not truly a lift which can only be done using plastic surgery, and perhaps, to an exponentially lesser degree and with limited success with a variety of "threadlifts." Again, our technique is to overlay the microcannula tip over the area to be enhanced to plan out the entry point for the Pilot needle to encompass the entirety of the area to be treated with the minimum of Pilot needle applications. We then simply enter and fan into the dermal-SQ junction after aspiration injecting retrograde and going forward with the Wiggle Progression Technique. Upon completion, we repeat the process at a 90 degree angle to complete the Long MicroCannula Double Cross-Hatched Fan Technique (LeeXX).

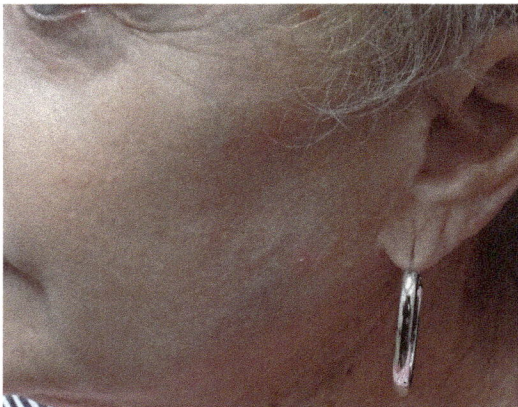

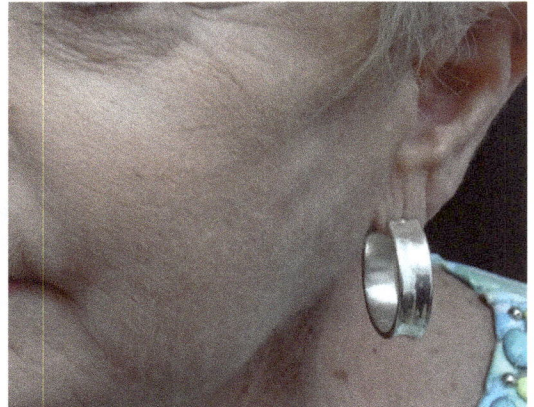

Crow's Feet
(orbicularis oculi) Technique

This traditional Botox Cosmetic® treatment area can also be injected with Juvederm Ultra Plus XC® for longer lasting results using the Long Microcannula Cross-Hatched Fan Technique (LeeXX).

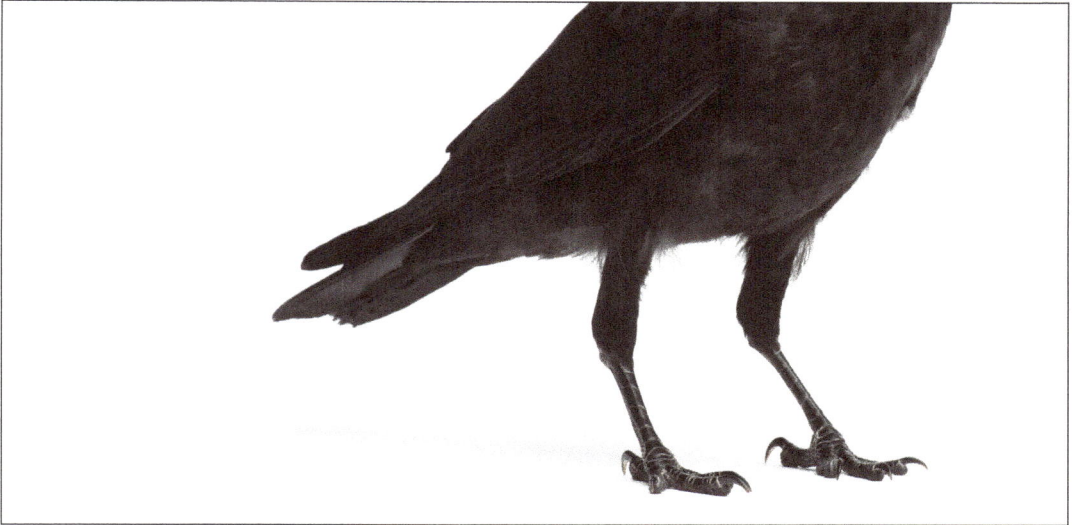

Cosmetic fillers may be a better and less expensive option, especially for those with large Crow's Feet muscles which may require excessive Botox Cosmetic® units which require treatment four times a year. Particular care must be taken to avoid the Transverse Facial and Zygomatico-orbital network of blood vessels in this area.

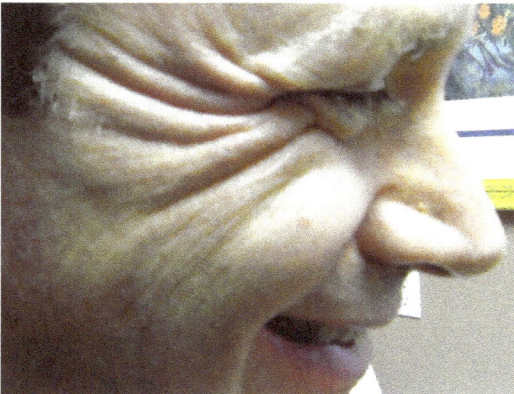

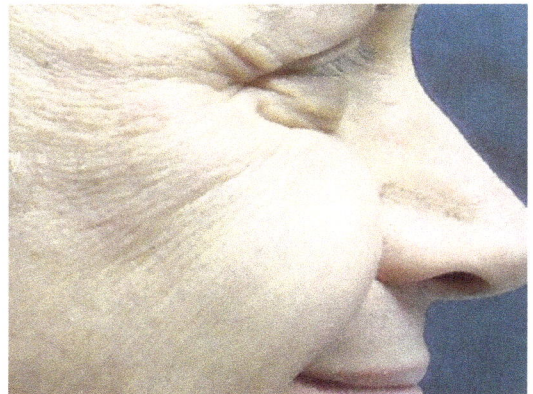

Before and After Juvederm® Treatment of Crow's Feet Using TSK STERiGLIDE Microcannula

Occipital Frontalis Technique

On the forehead, we use the Occipital Frontalis Technique to both static and dynamic wrinkles which is most aptly applied when Botox Cosmetic® cannot be used due to the likelihood of brow ptosis; the horizontal wrinkle is too proximal to the levator palpebrae superioris muscle with the risk of eyelid ptosis; the cost of Botox Cosmetic® is prohibitive due to the large size of the Occipital-Frontalis muscle; or Botox Cosmetic® is simply ineffective because the wrinkle is static instead of dynamic and can only be treated with cosmetic filler.

Note that I now classify this as a high risk area due the heightened risk of necrosis, embolism, and blindness from accidental injection of HA filler into a blood vessel, though I believe the risk to be less so than with the Glabella area. Consequently, I still treat this area with cosmetic injectable filler albeit only with pre-mapping of blood vessels using the AccuVein™ laser mapping system in conjunction with microcannula and aspiration. Again, I avoid any area mapped for blood vessels keeping in mind that the AccuVein™ system cannot be 100% accurate due to technological limitations of depth and precision.

The process is to place a Pilot needle at one end of a horizontal wrinkle, insert the microcannula using the Wiggle Progression Technique, and to repeat this sequentially until the entire length of the horizontal line is traversed, a process I call the "Pilot to Pilot Navigation." To facilitate this, I often map out the length of the microcannula directly over the line I am lifting to estimate where I will need to place the next Pilot hole in the succession. I then follow this linearly in "Pilot to Pilot Navigation."

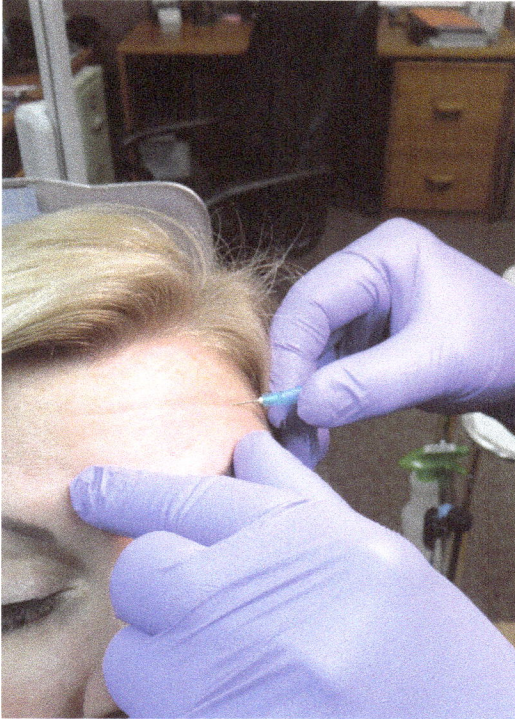
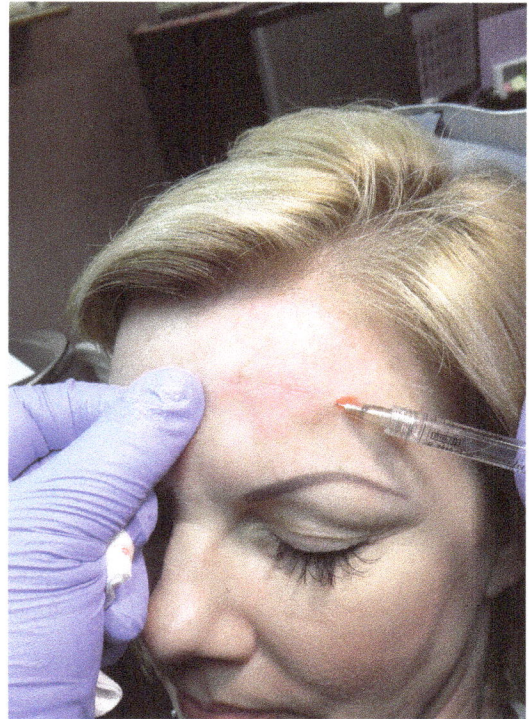

Pilot Insertion at Lateral Edge followed by Insertion to Entire Length of the Microcannula

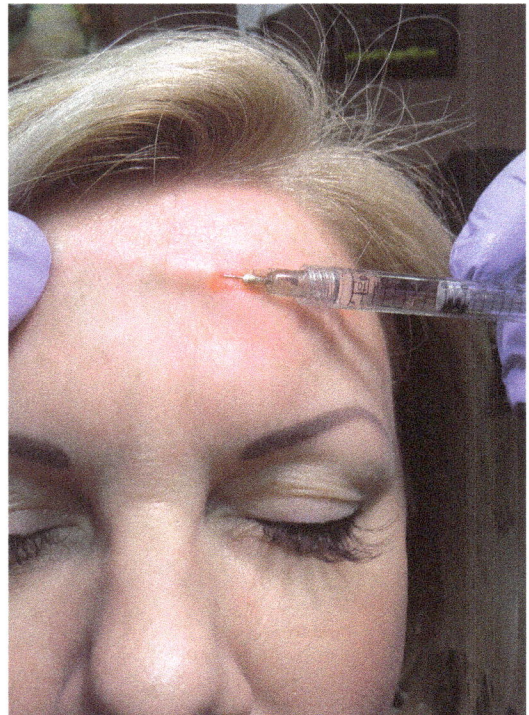
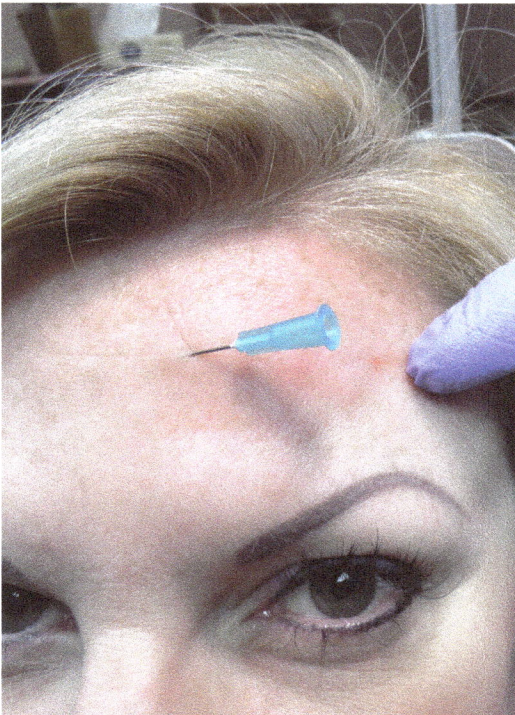

Mapping Placement of Next Pilot Needle at the Termination Point of the Last Microcannula Injection

Pilot to Pilot Navigation to Transverse Horizontal Occipital-Frontalis Wrinkle

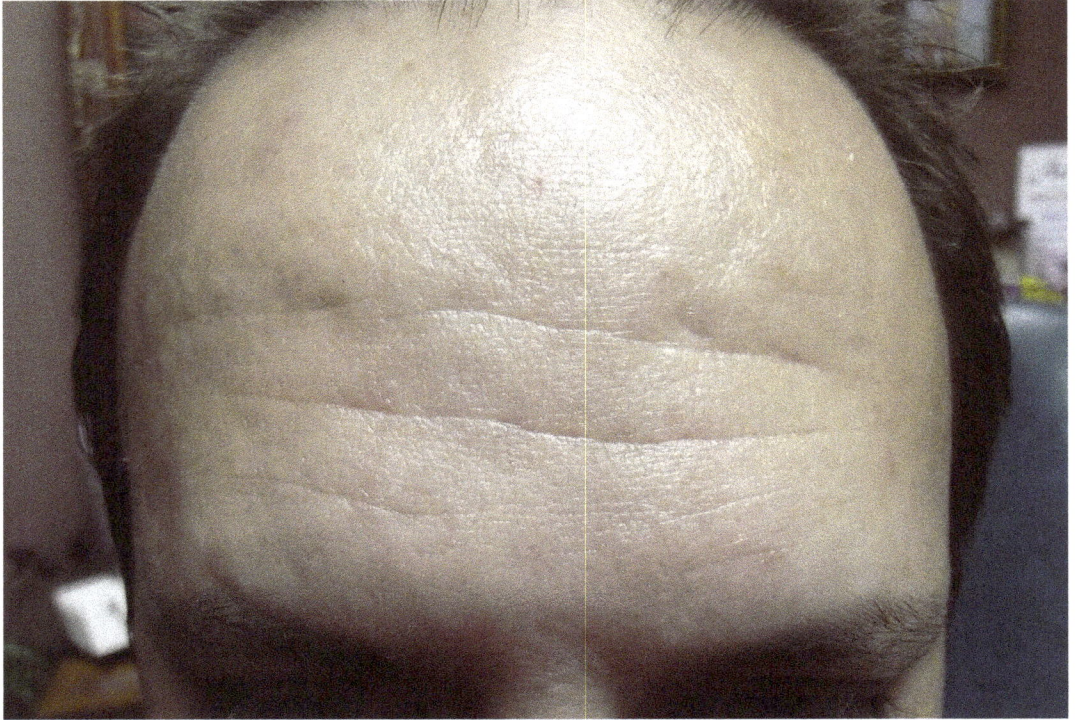

Before Frontalis Juvederm® Treatment Using TSK STERiGLIDE Microcannula

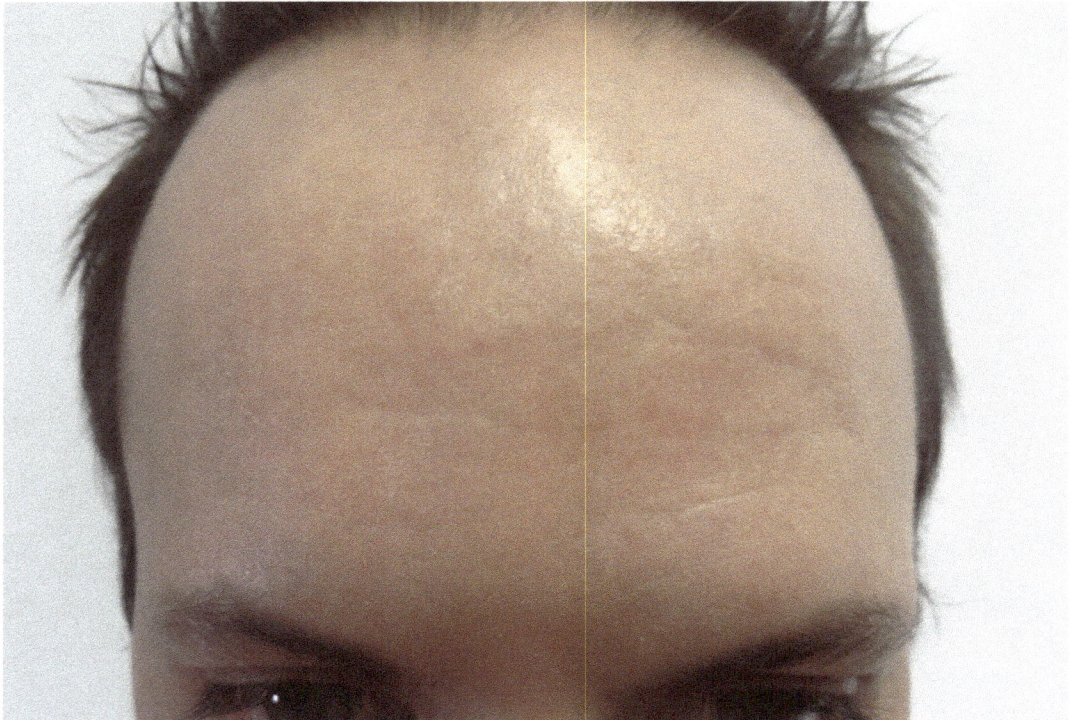

After Frontalis Juvederm® Treatment Using TSK STERiGLIDE Microcannula

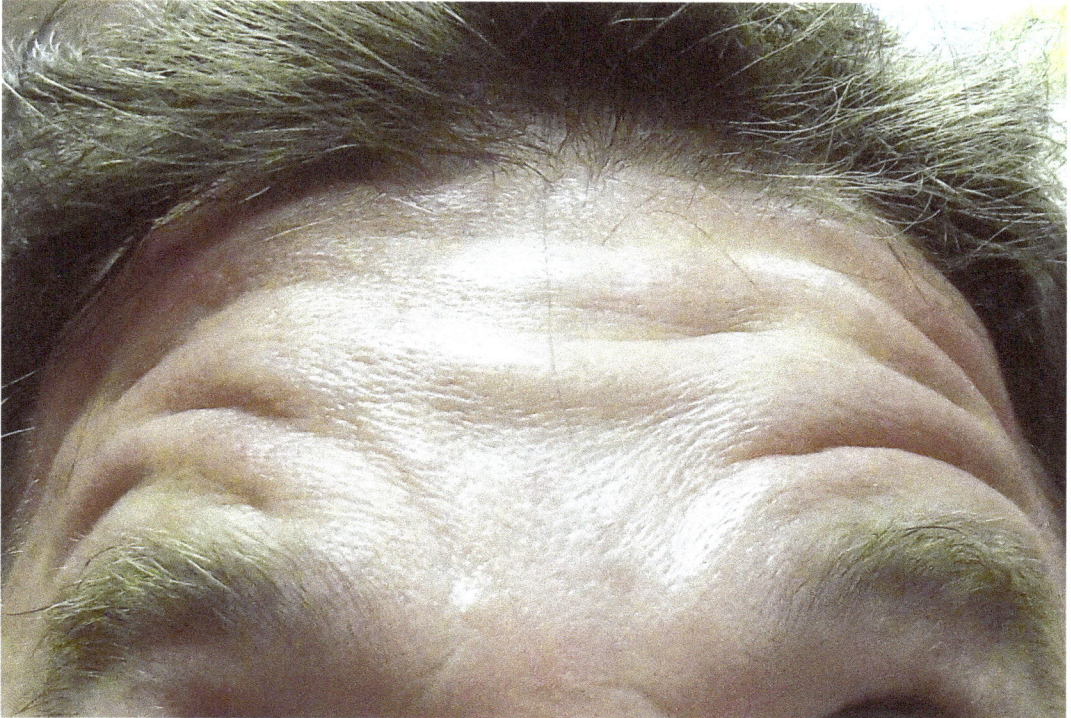

Pre-Juvederm® Frontalis

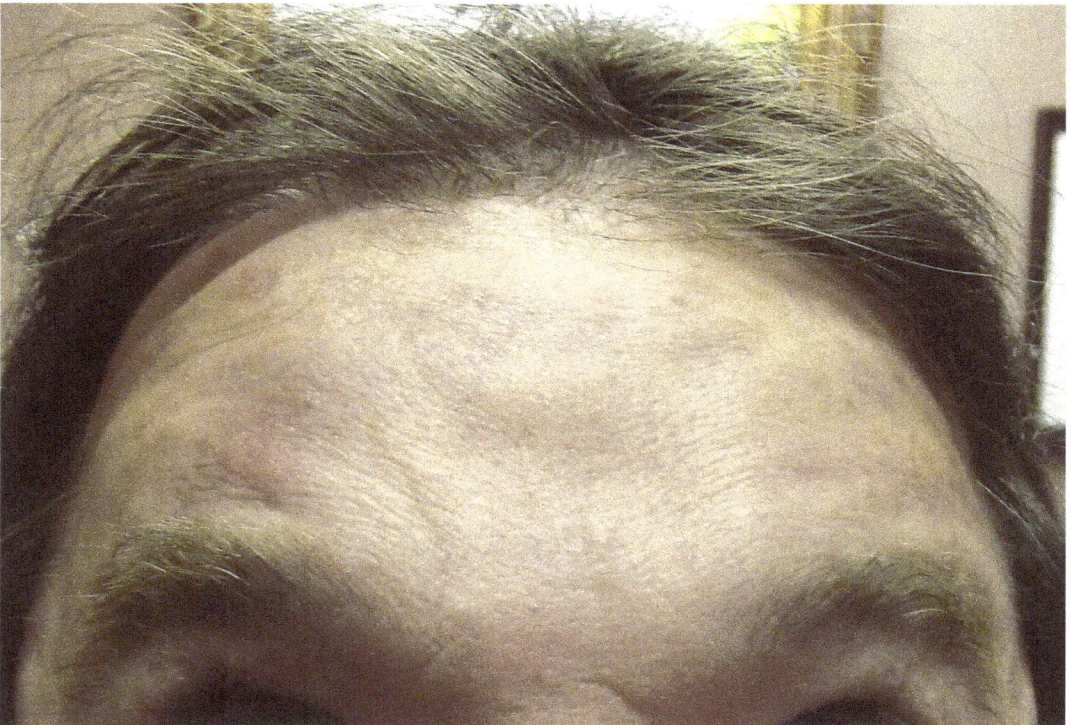

Dynamic Frontalis Wrinkles Injected With Juvederm Ultra Plus XC®

Temple Technique

This is a treatment area which is growing in popularity as we all age, which is also often overlooked as a foundation for renewal of the structure of the face. I have used both Sculptra® and Juvederm Ultra® with success in the temporal fossa, but again, treatment should be reserved only for experienced preceptorship trained injectors. Again, we use the AccuVein™ laser device to map out blood vessels to help prevent accidental intra-vascular injection.

With Juvederm Ultra,® I use the Long Microcannula Double Cross-Hatched Fan with the Wiggle Progression Technique only in the superficial plane of the dermal-SQ junction after mapping with AccuVein.™ I use particular care to aspirate and to inject slowly into the superficial subcutaneous tissue depression correction up to the temporal fusion line to prevent cannulation and resulting skin necrosis.

There is a tendency to swell with Juvederm,® especially in such a thin skin area, so placement must be deep enough to avoid visible lumping without any gaps in distribution.

Similarly, with Sculptra,® [20] I map with AccuVein™ then inject with a needle– not a microcannula – directly at a 90 degree angle into the mid-fossa just above the periosteum, aspirate back to check for back-flash, then bolus the Sculptra® slowly without fanning until I am at full correction of any skin depression. Then I massage it until it is completely smooth and have the patient do the traditional 5-5-5 Sculptra® massage technique of massaging the surrounding area vigorously for 5 minutes, 5 times a day, for 5 days in a row.

Note that it is especially important that massage encompass the entire surrounding area and that it be done precisely as directed for this minimal time, or a Sculptra® nodule may form, commonly at the periphery.

While Galderma's 5-5-5 massage technique is not evidenced based, nevertheless I have seen nodules formed by Sculptra® in the Temporal Fossa and I would much rather take this precaution if there is any chance at all that it may reduce nodule formation.

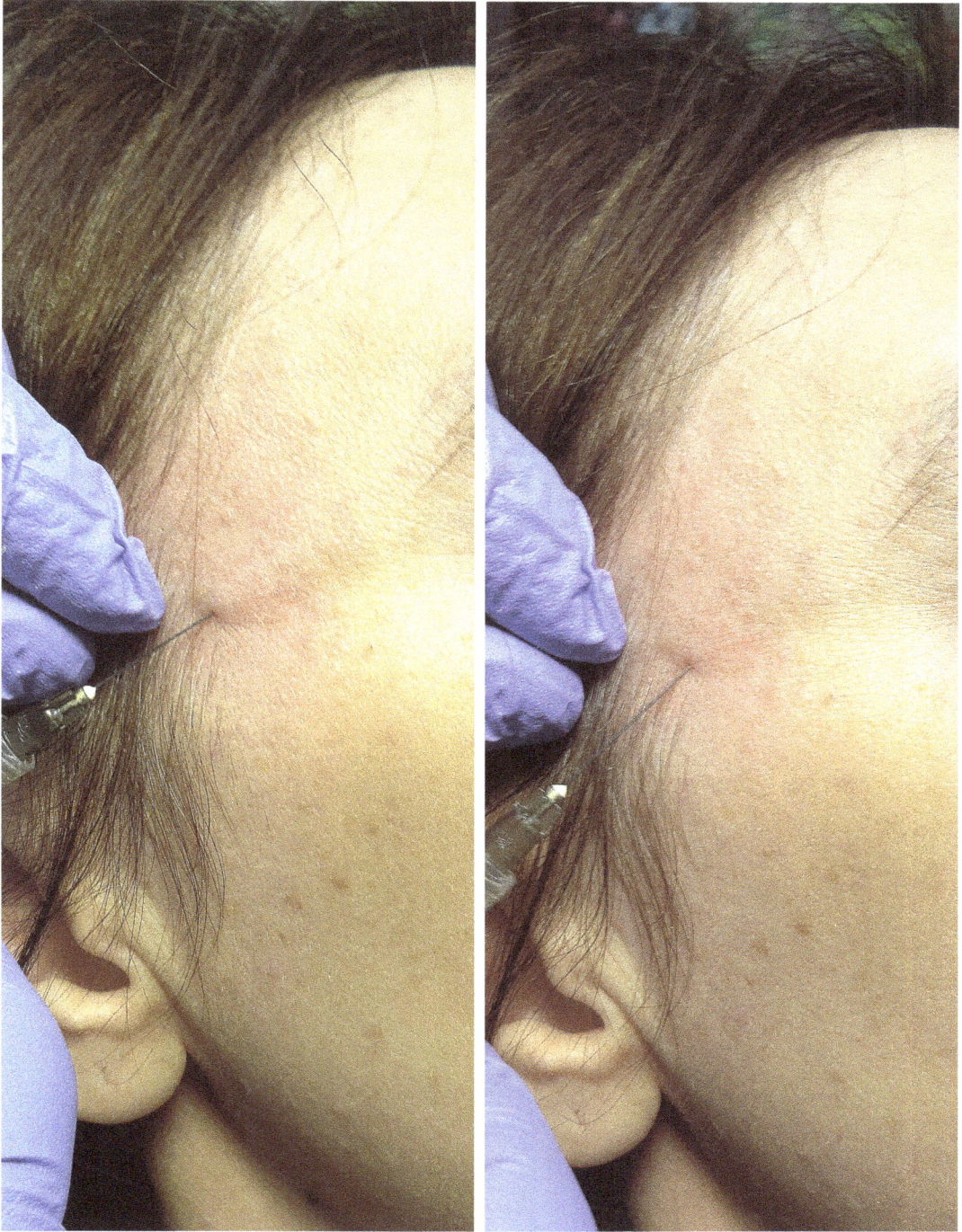

Juvederm® Injection Into Temporal Fossa

Glabella TentLee Technique

The glabella is the confluence of the right corrugator muscle, the procerus muscle, and the left corrugator muscle between the eyes which may give rise to the connotation of anger, even when no such emotion exists. Classically, we find two or more vertical wrinkles present which are really the junction between these muscles, often characterized as the "elevens," for their appearance. This is a high risk injection area where blindness and stroke[17, 34] have been reported after the accidental cannulation of small caliber vessels branching from supratrochlear arteries which have minimal collateral circulation. The resulting necrosis often leads to ulceration and ultimately scarring.

With the recent reports of increasing complications of injecting cosmetic fillers into the glabella from accidental cannulation of blood vessels, I am far more selective of who I treat here with cosmetic injectable fillers because of the risk of necrosis, embolization, infarction, and even blindness – however small – in this high risk area.

Glabella *TentLee Technique*

Our protocol is to view and map the blood vessels in the glabella area under the AccuVein™ [29] laser device to see if there is any apparent overlap of skin laxity lines with blood vessels. If the area appears to be relatively avascular, we will slowly inject a tiny amount of filler using microcannula by "tenting" the treatment area upwards with the microcannula tip maintaining constant pressure with the dermal-SQ junction, what we call our *Glabella TentLee Technique.*

If there is a blood vessel nearby, we slowly inject about a millimeter or two away – adjacent to it – and gently massage the filler into the adjacent area. Our protocol is to only inject here after pre-mapping with AccuVein,™ "tenting" the blunt tip of microcannula upwards, then aspiration followed by slow, low-volume retrograde injection with the Wiggle Progression technique. We use aspiration regardless of the question of its effectiveness – as this may, or may not, add additional safety to treatment in a high risk area, but certainly can do no harm.

We also advocate treatment of minor skin laxity in the glabella with laser or other energy skin tightening treatments often in combination with a series of microneedling and Platelet-Rich Plasma **(PRP)** treatment.

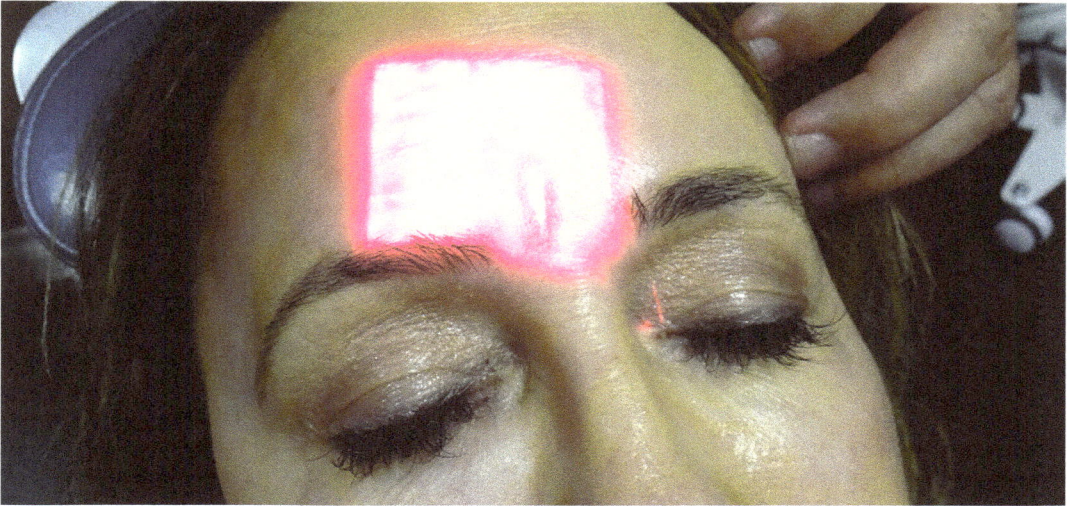

AccuVein™ illustrates the blood vessel previously invisible to the injector

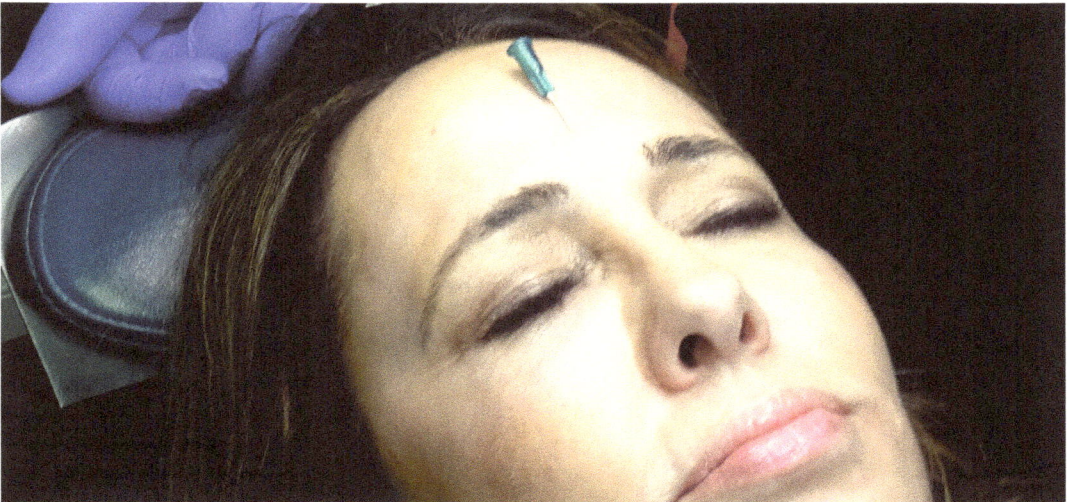

Pilot Needle Placement is from above the patient for Glabella TentLee Technique

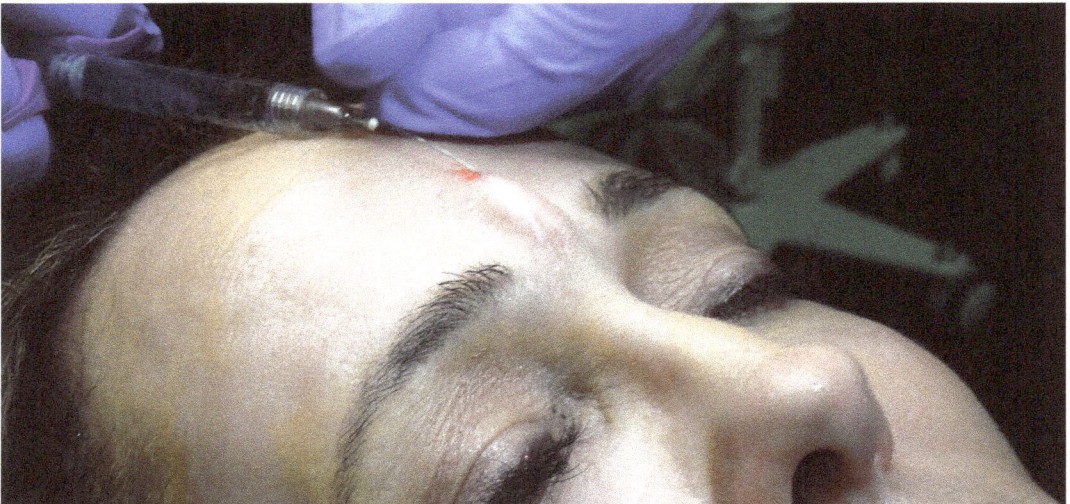

Microcannula tip is "Tented" upwards; injection is ~1.0 mm lateral to white vascular marker

Alternatively, the Carruthers[4] report great success and safety by injection into the lower medial aspect of the Glabella to the periosteum, concurrent with manual massage superiorly to recreate the foundation of the Glabella. Their selection that this relatively avascular area is the key to their protocol may ultimately make it the standard for the glabella area.

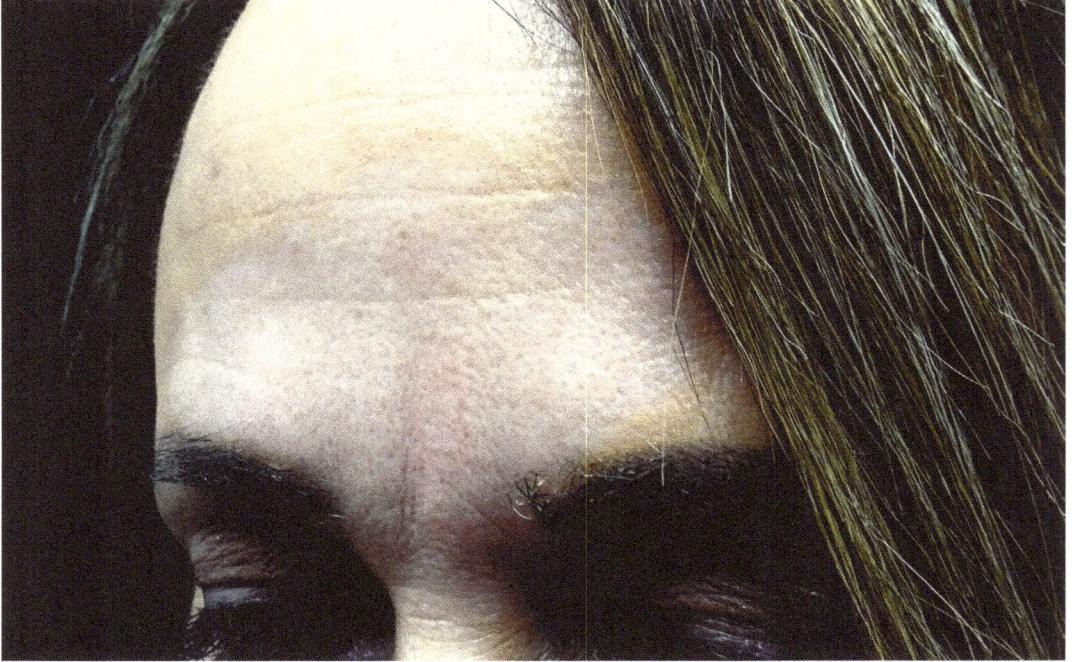

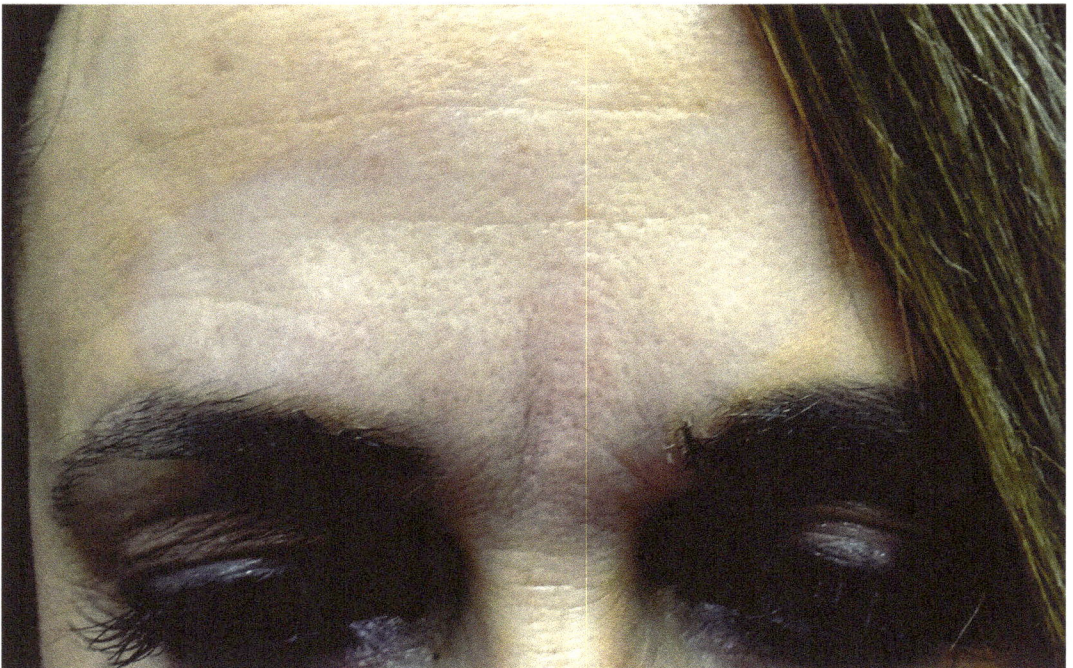

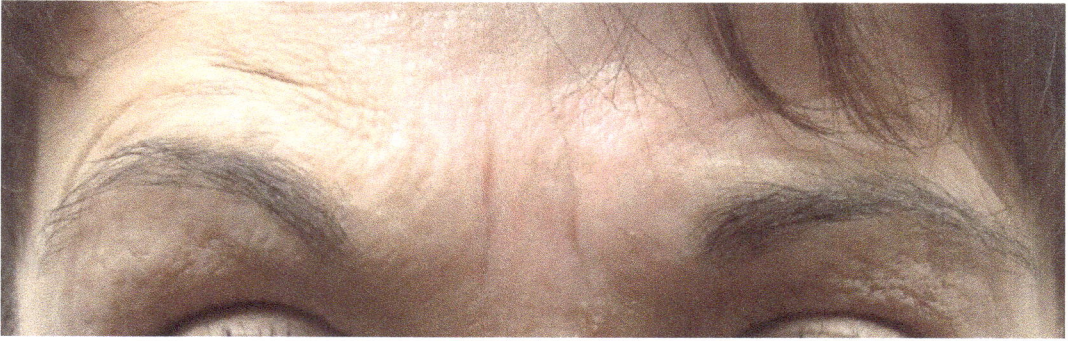

Pre-Glabella (The "Elevens") Treatment with Cosmetic Fillers

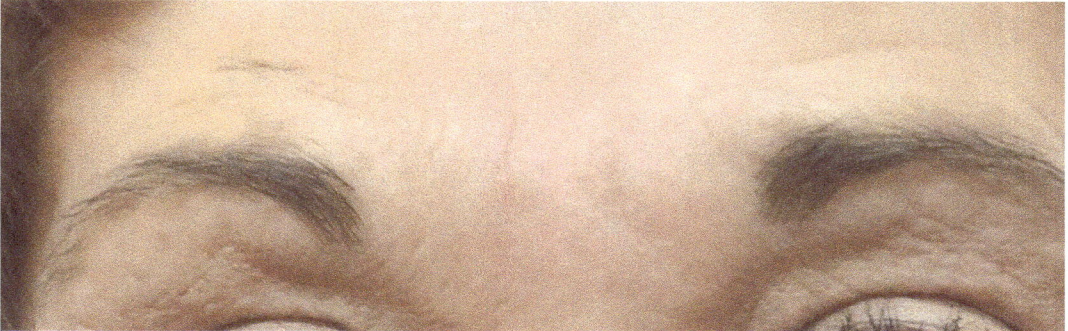

Post-Glabella Initial Treatment with Cosmetic Fillers

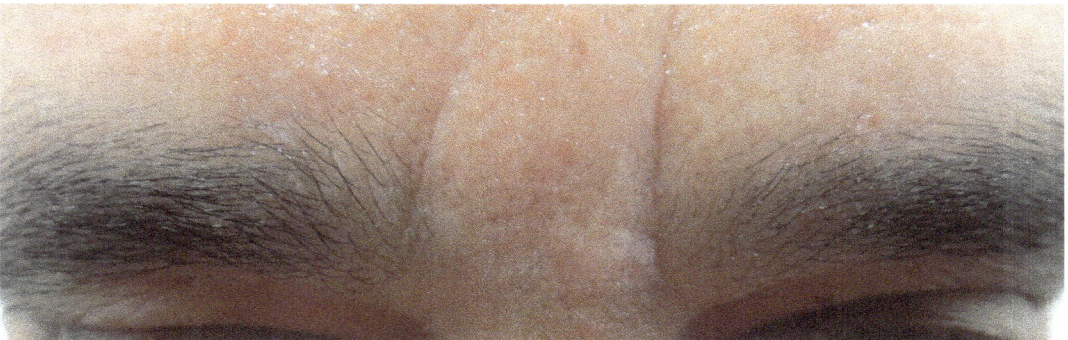

Glabella Static Wrinkle Treatment Using Juvederm® with STERiGLIDE Microcannula

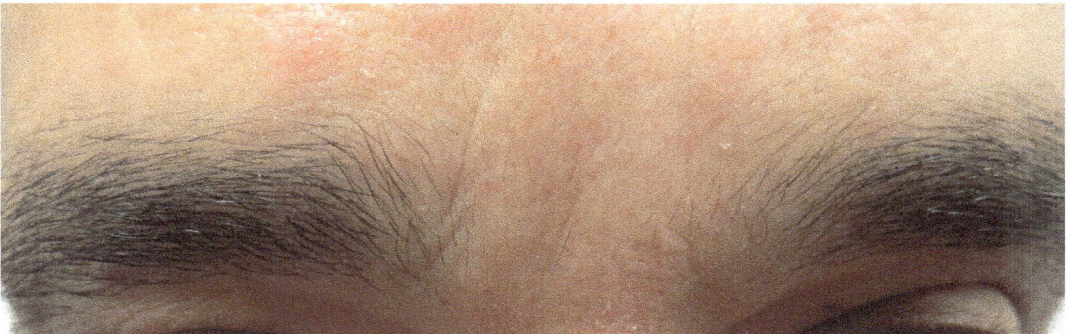

NOTES

Microcannula Body Techniques

Neck Technique

Microcannula may also be used to inject cosmetic fillers into neck wrinkles, but a great deal of extra care must be taken to avoid the plethora of blood vessels endemic in this area. Our procedure is to use the AccuVein™ to illuminate the most prominent blood vessels and a surgical marker to delineate them as areas to be avoided. I use the 1½" microcannula to inject very superficially with tenting the tip of the microcannula to the dermal-SQ junction to avoid any cannulation of deeper blood vessels. Before injection, I aspirate back on the syringe to further reduce the risk of injecting into a blood vessel. Then I use "Pilot to Pilot Navigation" to repeat the process until the entire length of the desired wrinkle is completed.

Sculpting cosmetic filler in the neck is particularly difficult because there are no bony or hard structures against which to mold the filler, so while good results may be obtained, we are currently testing other non-surgical modalities to better treat this area.

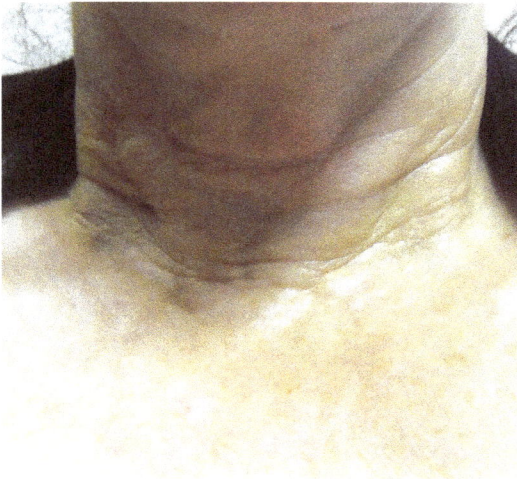

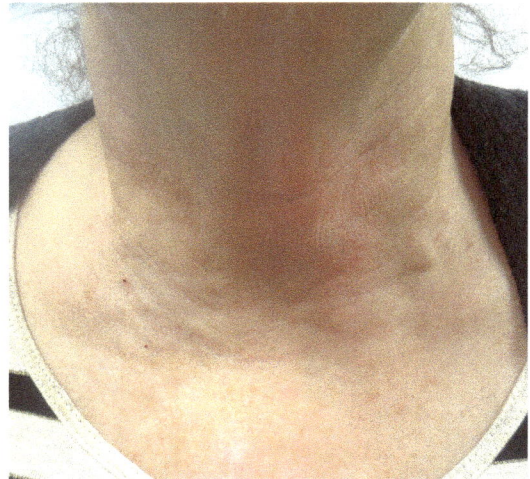

Before and After Neck Treatment Using Juvederm® with TSK STERiGLIDE Microcannula

Chest
(or Chest Wrinkle) Technique

Patients with large breasts or with too much sun damage may have unsightly wrinkles in the cleavage or décolleté between the breasts from excessive skin laxity. I originally placed the Pilot hole superior to the chest wrinkle, or what I term the "Chrinkle," but found working around my patient's head difficult, so I now place the Pilot using the inferior approach injecting at the base of the Chrinkle. I use a 27 Gage 1½" microcannula with Juvederm Ultra Plus XC,® and occasionally with Juvederm Voluma® or Restylane Lyft® using the Long Microcannula Double Cross-Hatched Fan Technique (LeeXX).

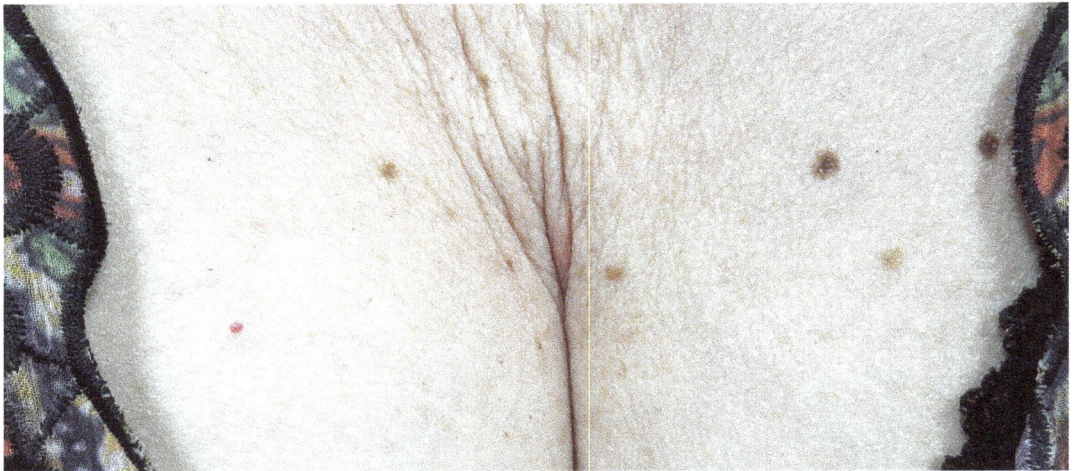

Chrinkle Treatment Using Juvederm Ultra Plus® and Voluma®
with TSK STERiGLIDE Microcannula

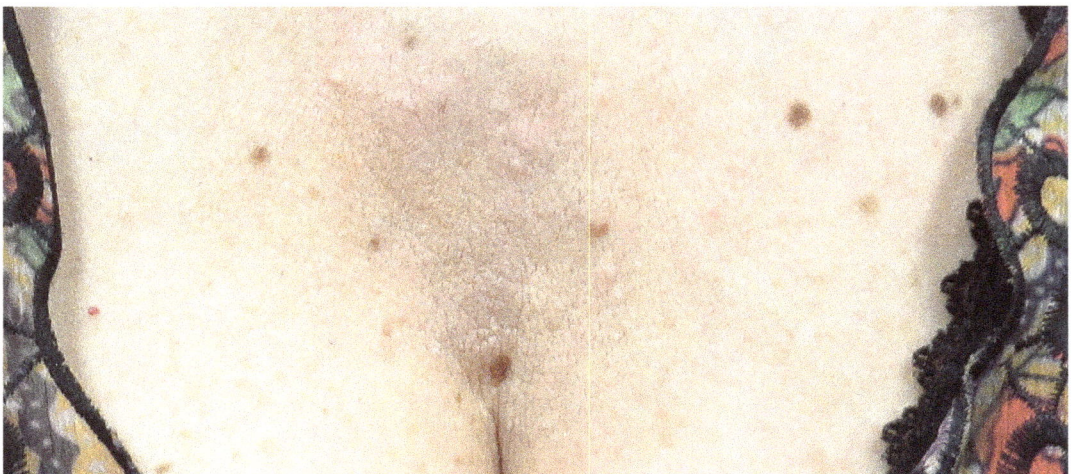

Hand Technique

Often, it is the hands that give away one's age but now, we can inject cosmetic fillers such as Restylane Lyft® or Radiesse® (Off-Label) to hide the unsightly extensor surface blood vessels.

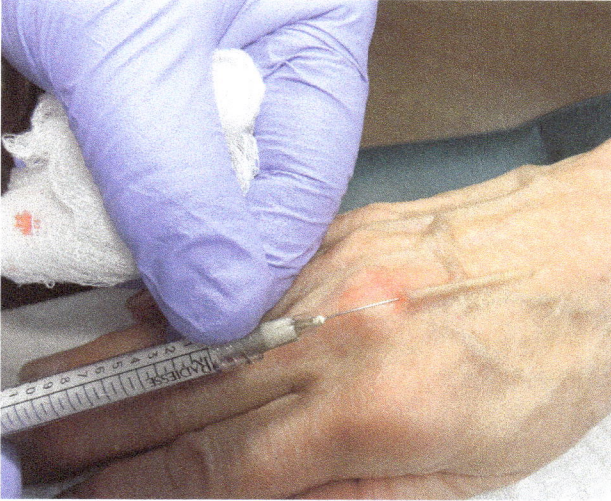

The microcannula technique on the dorsum of the hand is to place the Pilot into the hand just proximal to the MCP joints and to use entry at either one (3rd phalange for smaller hands) or two portals (in line with the 2nd and 4th phalanges for larger hands) to encompass the entire extensor surface of the hand.

Radiesse® Injection with TSK STERiGLIDE Microcannula Glides Over Vein

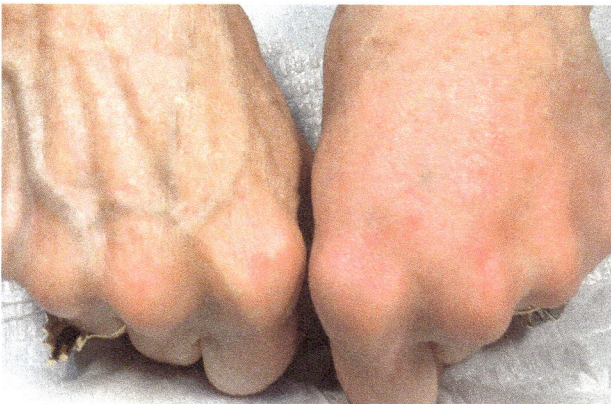

As you can see, with a little finesse, the microcannula can literally glide over blood vessels without penetration using the Wiggle Progression Technique with excellent results using the 1½" microcannula.

Left Hand Immediately After Radiesse® Injection Using TSK STERiGLIDE Microcannula

Our observation is that Restylane Lyft® – which is On-Label in this area but not with microcannula – typically requires 3-5 syringes for adequate hand extensor surface volume replacement for most women patients however, Radiesse® typically only requires two 1.5 cc syringes, making this a far more economical procedure for our aesthetic patients.

Buttocks & Body Techniques

Although we typically think of cosmetic fillers for injection of the face, I use it Off-Label in other appropriate body areas. Here application is made to the upper thigh after overly aggressive liposuction and in the buttocks for a lipoatrophy defect (to correct Kenalog® steroid injection a physician did here for allergic rhinitis).

The Long Microcannula Double Cross-Hatched Fan (LeeXX) Technique was used with Juvederm Ultra Plus.®

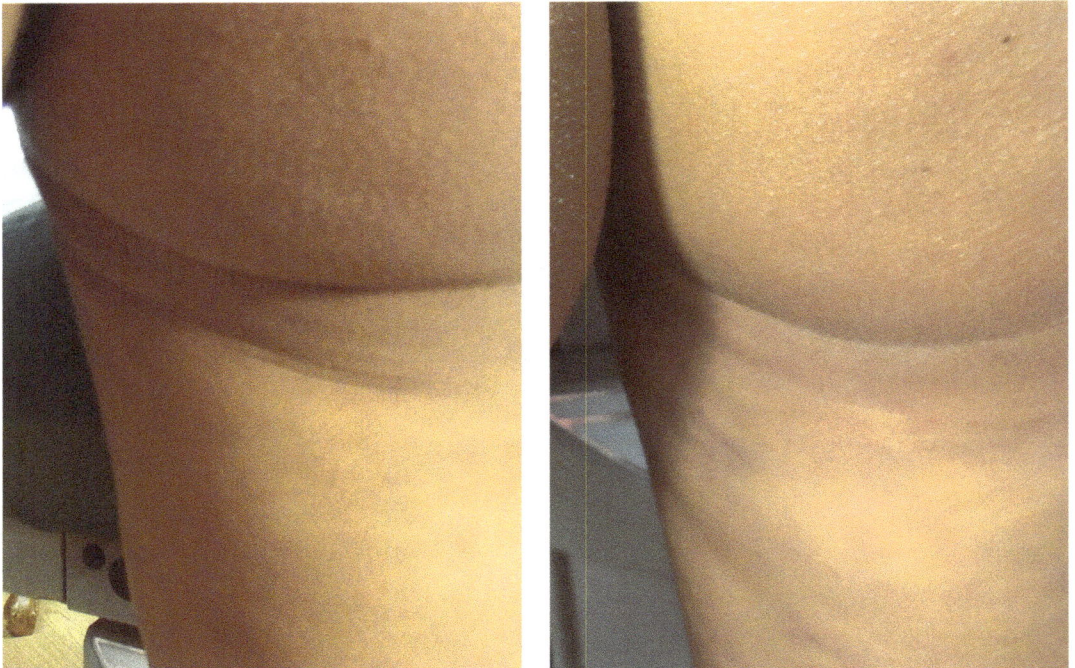

Cosmetic Filler Using the Long Microcannula Double Cross-Hatched Fan to Correct Excessive Liposuction.

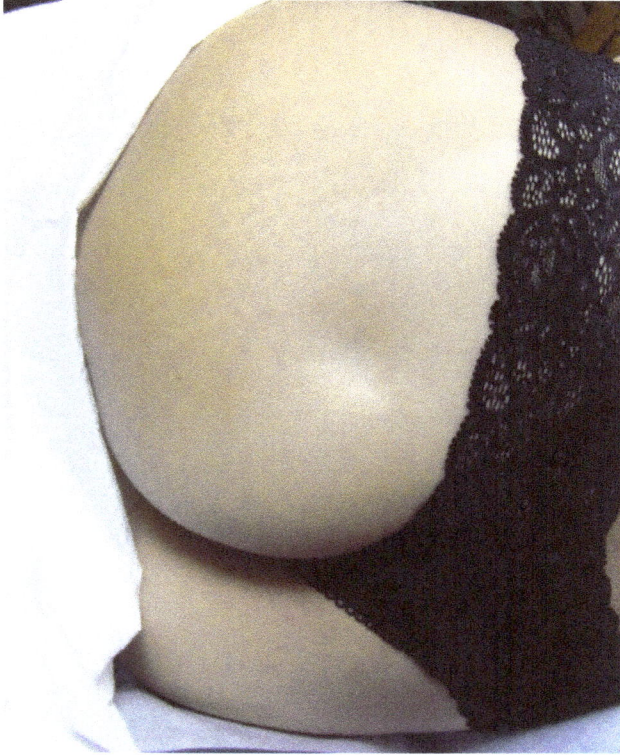

Pre/Post Treatment Left Buttock Lipoatrophy Defect Treatment with Juvederm®
Using TSK STERiGLIDE Microcannula

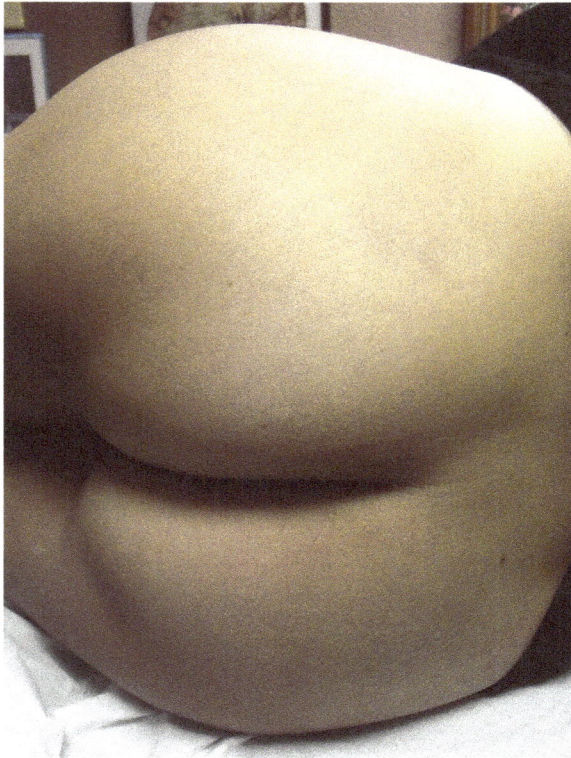

NOTES

Combination Treatments for Cosmetic Fillers

With Microneedling and Platelet-Rich Plasma (PRP)

Traditionally we typically do just a single treatment followed by a series of additional sessions. However, since 2015 (credit Dr. Tess Mauricio), we found that a multi-treatment combination in single session minimizes down time, incorporates other mechanisms of action, and appears to increase the potential for maximal success. The secret is to find "The Right Stuff" in a combination of minimally invasive aesthetic procedures done in one session which promotes synergy.

Our 2019 sequence is 1) inject cosmetic filler using AccuVein™ [29] Navigation, Mapping, and microcannula with the Wiggle Progression, 2) draw and spin Eclipse Platelet-Rich Plasma[53] (PRP), and 3) then treat the skin with microneedling[49, 50] using PRP.

PRP are platelets and human growth factors drawn from the patient's own peripheral (usually antecubital) blood vessel, then super-concentrated after centrifuge separation. PRP recently obtained FDA approval for use in joints to accelerate healing with orthopedic surgery,[51, 52] but is increasingly being used "Off-Label" for many other applications such as aesthetic medicine,[53, 54] though specific FDA indication and applicable research is still pending.

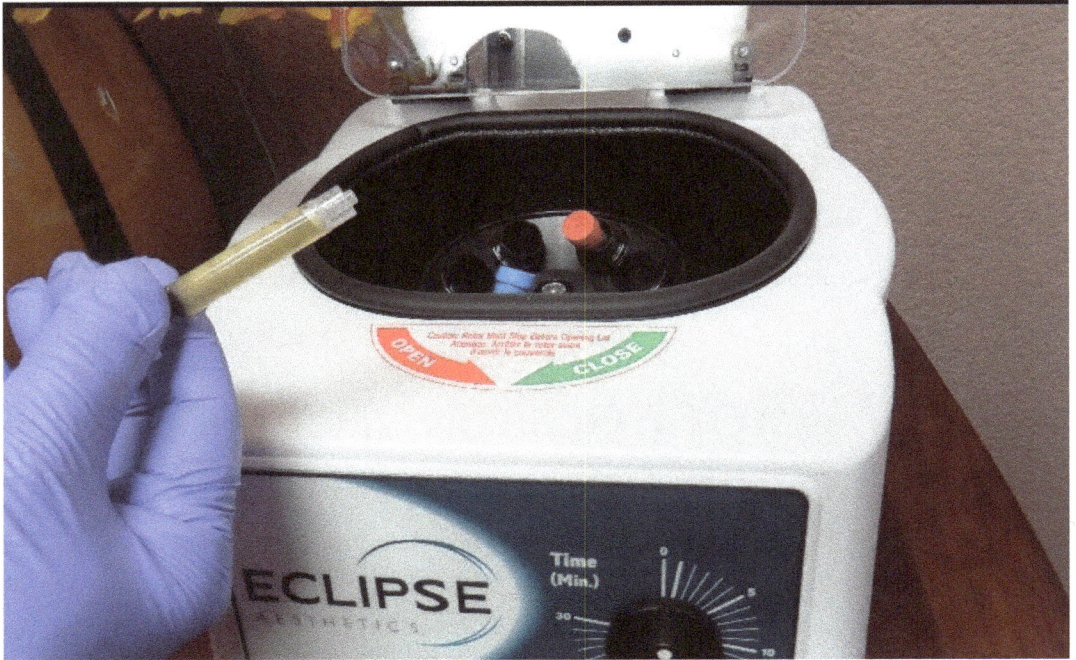

PRP Concentrated After Centrifuge; MicroNeedling to Stimulate Collagen Production

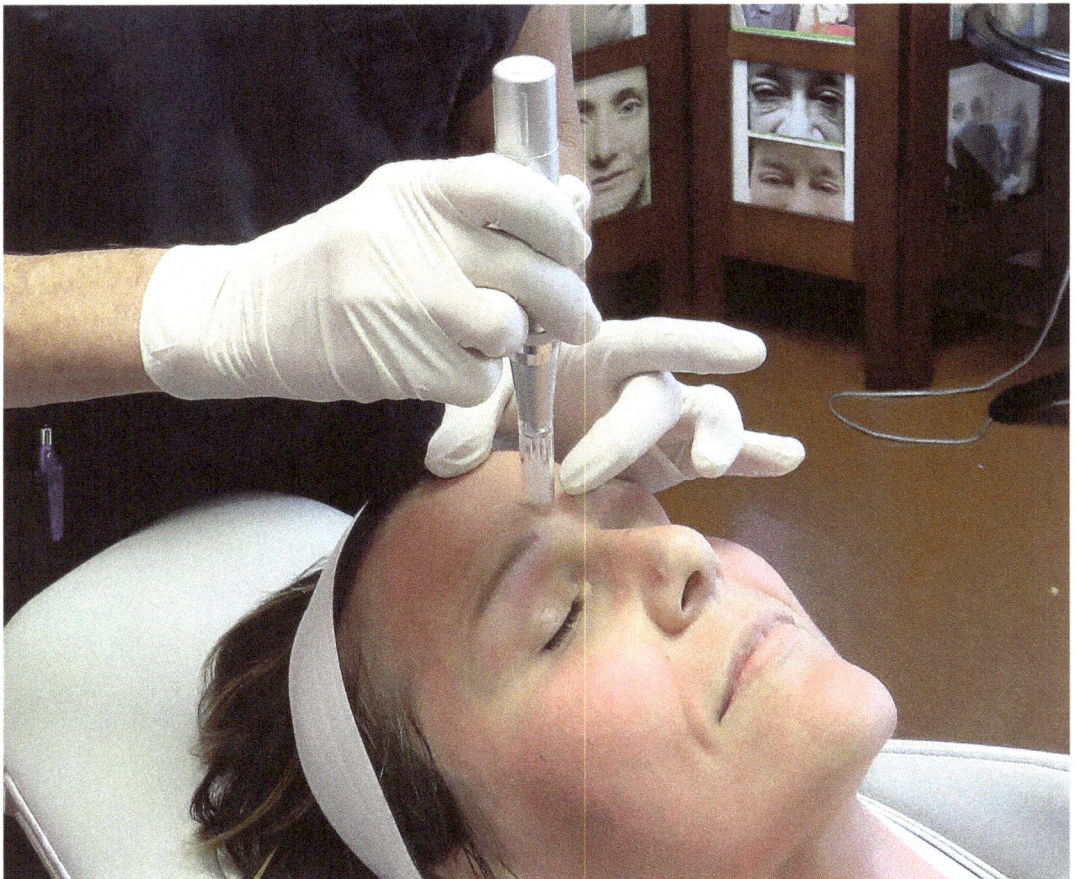

Automated Micro-Needling[49, 50] (also known as Collagen Induction Therapy or CIT) is the use of a mechanical device which vibrates tiny needles at high speed to penetrate the skin and create controlled micro-injuries in order to stimulate the production of collagen and elastin. This is used to treat the appearance of fine lines and acne scars to improve the skin's overall appearance. Correspondingly, this also creates superficial micro-channels (credit: Gordon H. Sasaki, MD, FACS) through the skin which temporarily may enhance the absorption of Platelet-Rich Plasma (PRP), topical gels, creams, and serums to stimulate even greater improvement in the appearance of the skin.

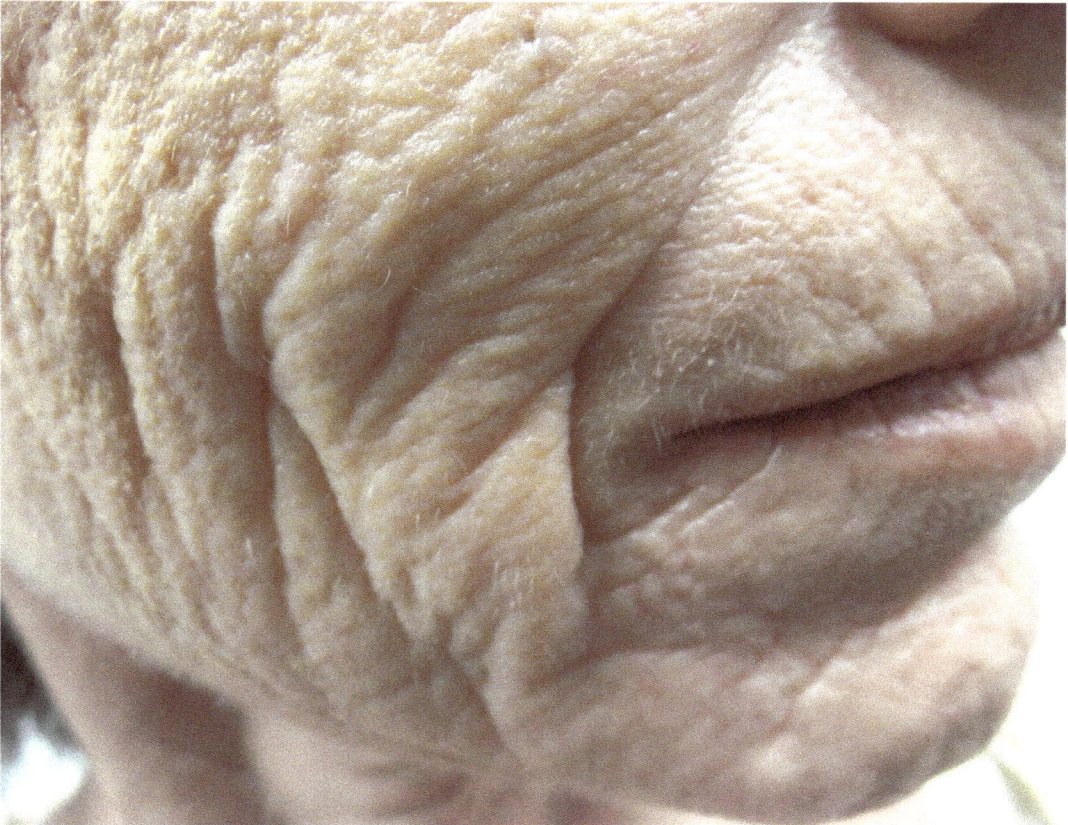

Close-Up Patient Prior to Combined Treatment

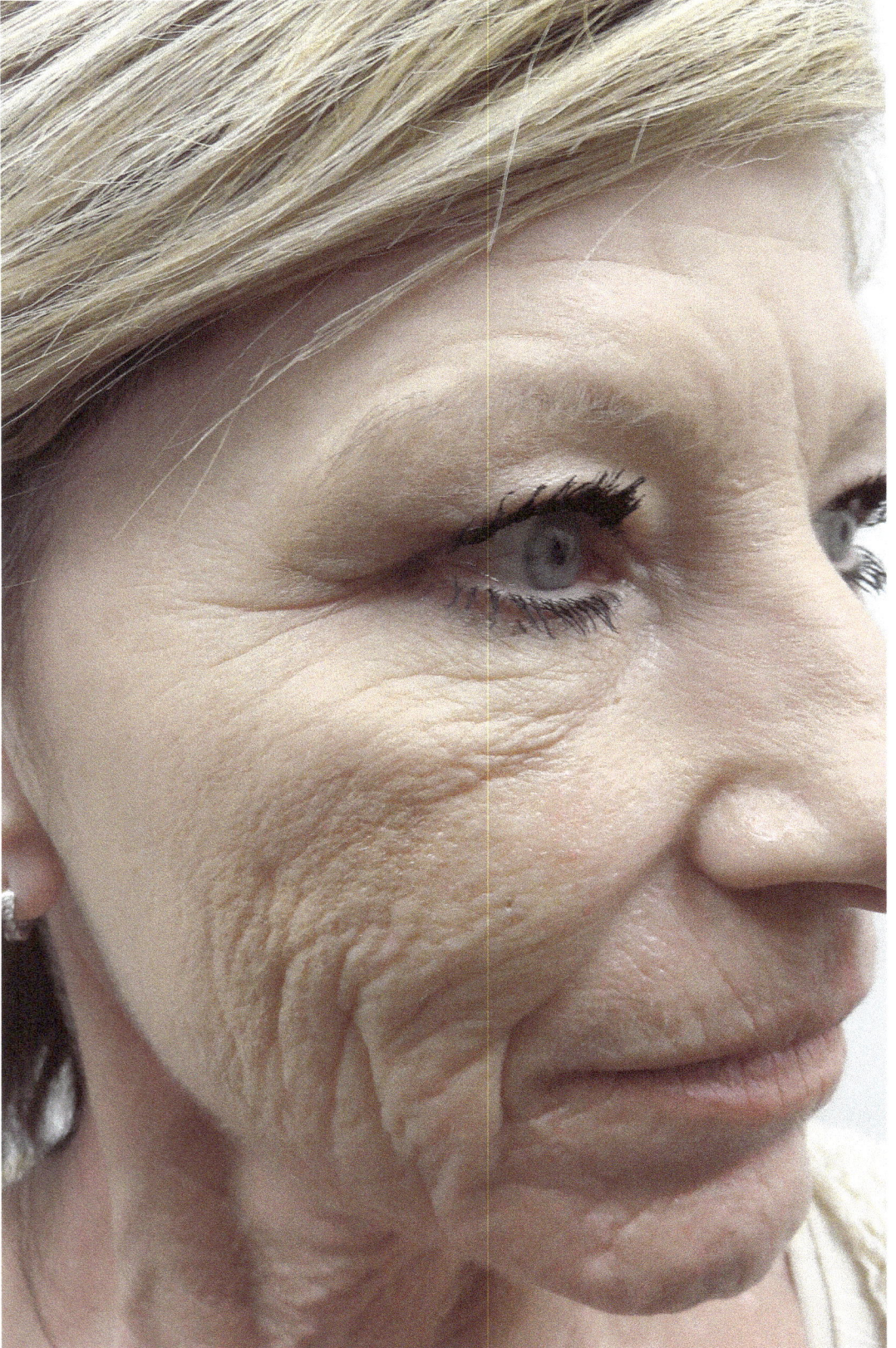

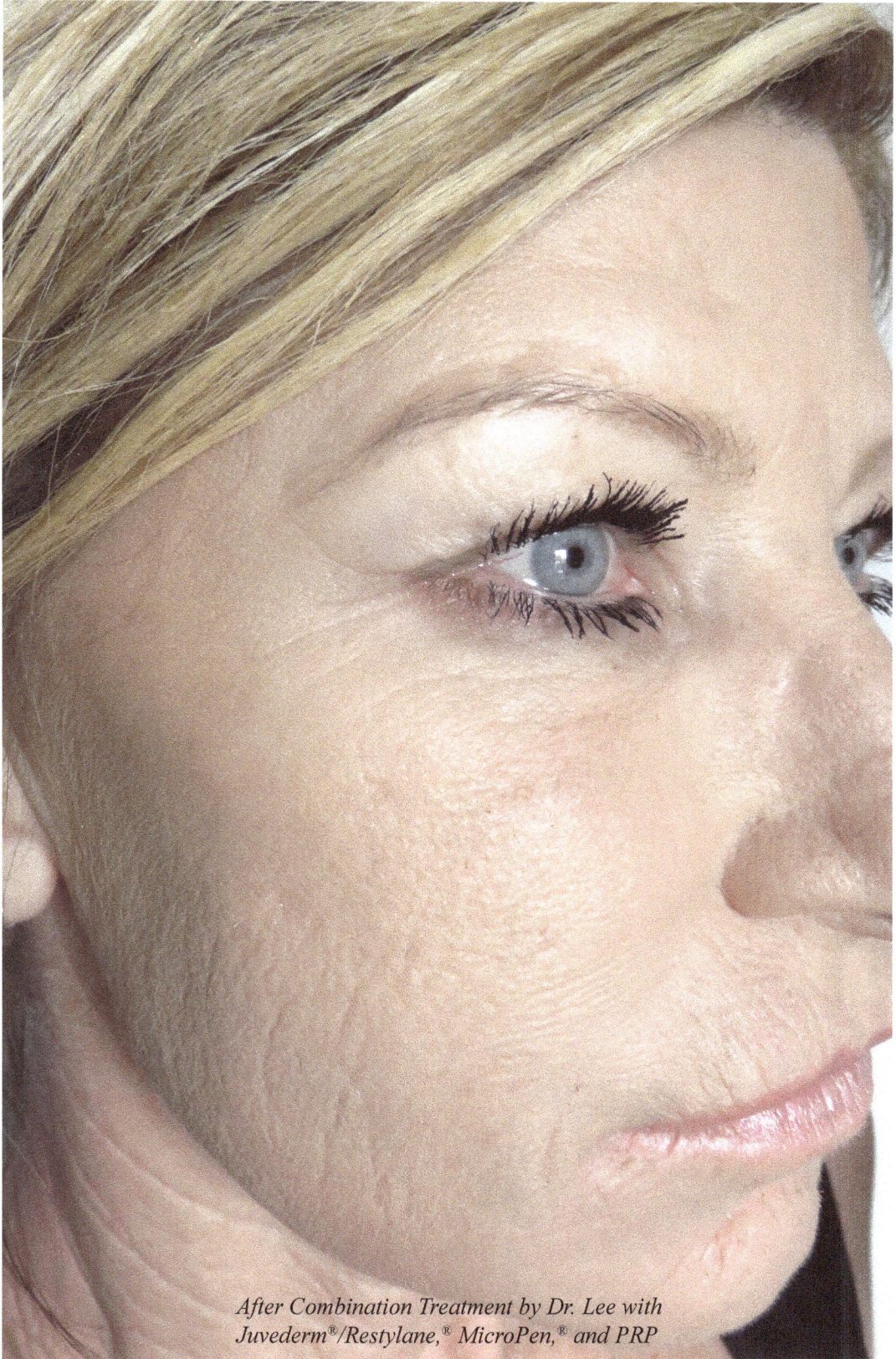

After Combination Treatment by Dr. Lee with
Juvederm®/Restylane,® MicroPen,® and PRP

With Radio Frequency, MicroNeedling, and PRP

Skinfinity RF® 55 is a fractional ablative radio frequency device used for skin tightening and skin resurfacing of the face, neck, and body to reduce wrinkles, fine lines, rosacea, acne scars, and stretch marks. It also assists with the correction of uneven skin tone and texture while simultaneously promoting collagen production. Our preferred sequence (credit: Tess Mauricio, MD, FAAD) is 1) inject cosmetic filler using AccuVein™ mapping and microcannula, 2) draw and spin Eclipse PRP, 3) do Skinfinity RF,® and 4) do microneedling using PRP. Note that the combination of these technologies is an Off-Label application and must be indicated as such in informed consent.

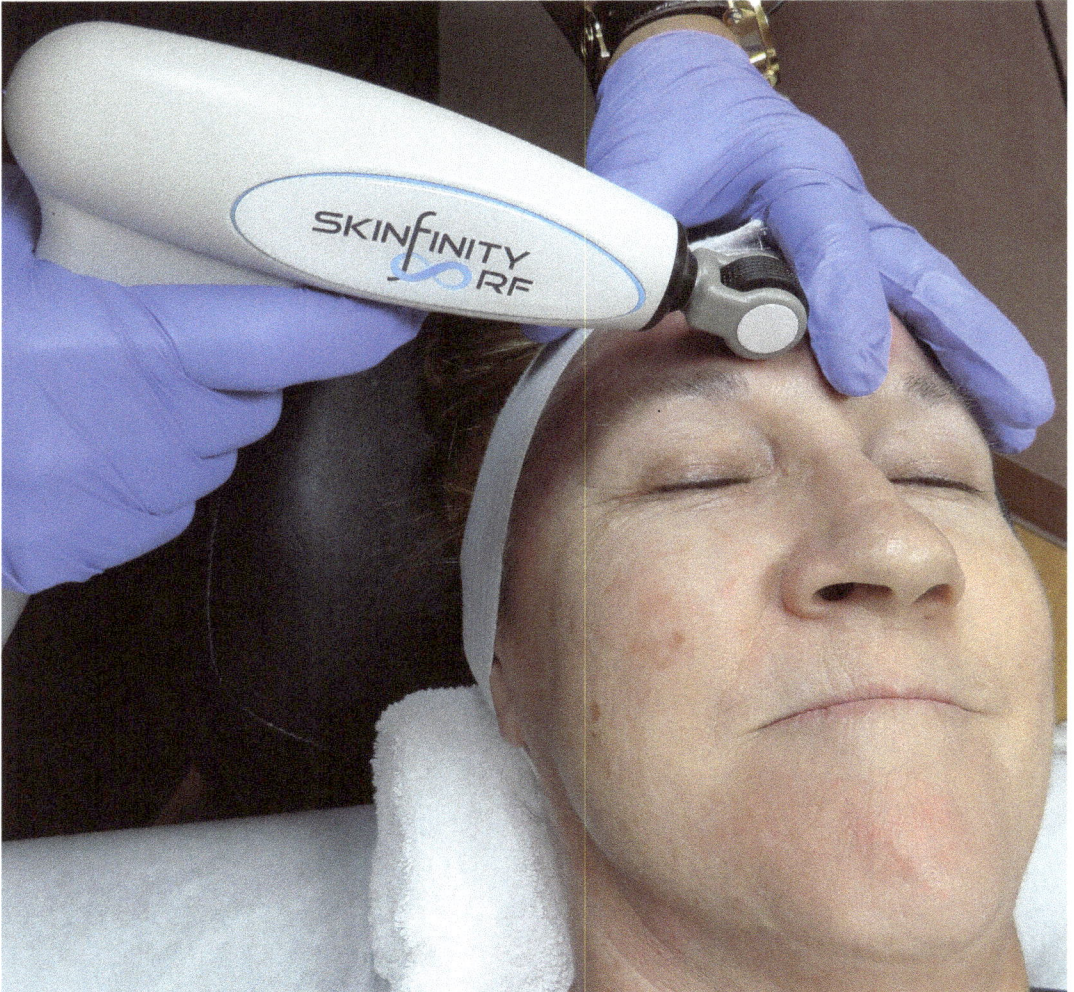

Alternatively, other RF/combination devices, lasers, or energy technology may be used in place of Skinfinity RF if deemed equivalent by each individual practitioner, however I suggest careful consideration of Fitzpatrick Skin Types and conduction of a test spot for the use of alternative technology.

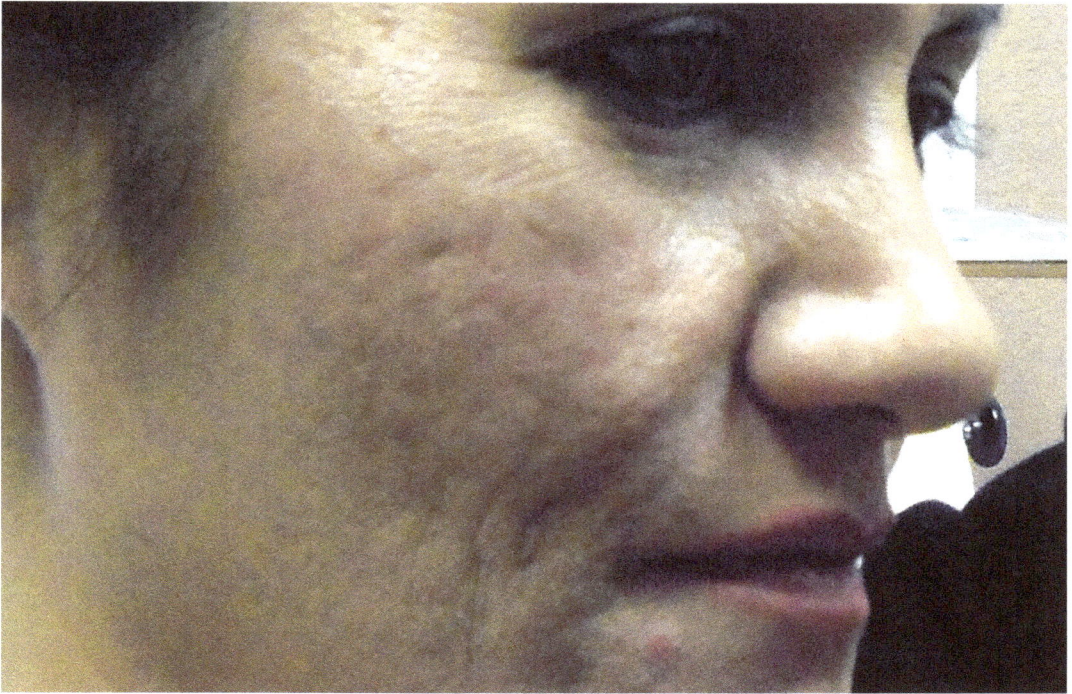

Pre/Post Combined Treatment with Juvederm,® Skinfinity RF,® MicroPen,® and PRP

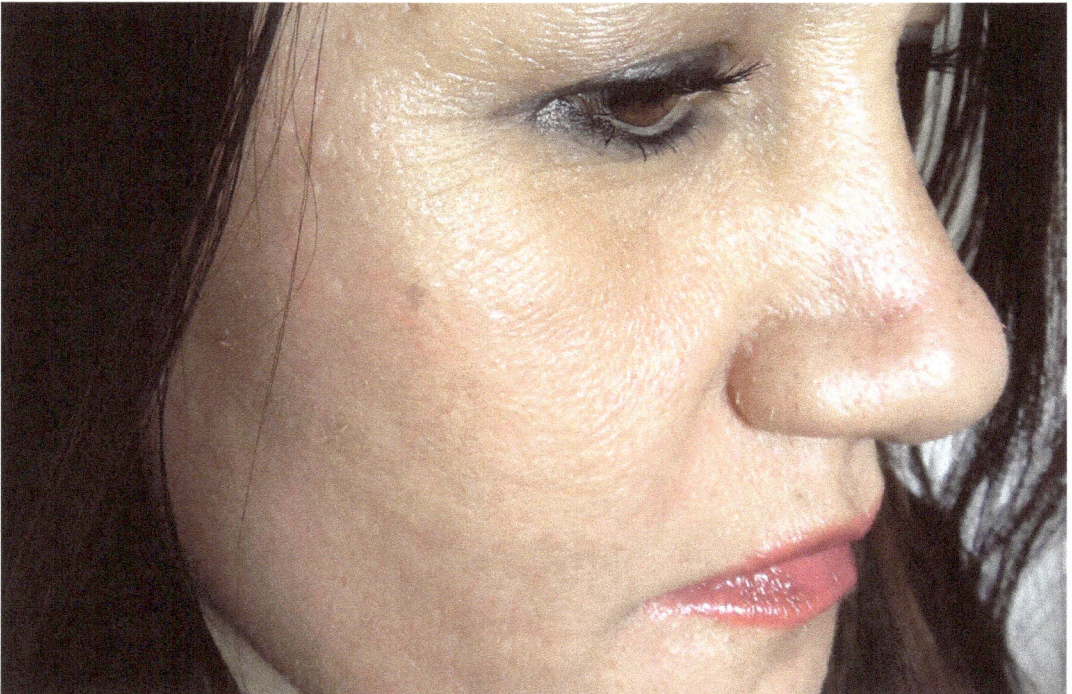

NOTES

Hyaluronic Acid Filler Safety

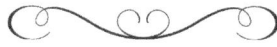

~~~~~~

Hyaluronidase Enzyme

Why Is Hyaluronic Acid (HA) Enzyme Important?

Anyone doing cosmetic injectable HA fillers can always add more filler if the amount injected is insufficient. But what happens if we accidentally inject too much – or worse, inject inadvertently into a blood vessel which can cause necrosis or emboli? Fortunately, the enzyme for hyaluronic acid, hyaluronidase,[22, 48, 56, 57] exists and is available in the USA, albeit use for reversal of HA filler is decidedly an Off-Label, or unapproved FDA application without substantiating research.

What Is It?

Hyaluronidase[58] is an enzyme which causes extracellular hydrolysis of hyaluronic acid which lowers viscosity, and correspondingly increases tissue permeability. The hyaluronidase FDA indications to date are only to speed dispersion and delivery of medications in ophthalmology, subcutaneous absorption of fluids by hypodermoclysis, and resorption of radiopaque agents. Animal-derived manufactured brands include Vitrase (ISTA) and the Synthetic (recombinant or rDNA) hyaluronidase in the USA is Hylenex[47] (Halozyme Therapeutics).

Contraindications and Precautions

Hylenex recombinant is contraindicated in patients with known hypersensitivity to hyaluronidase or any components of Hylenex recombinant. Precautions must be taken to prevent the spread of localized infection because increased dispersion will spread infection. Hylenex does contain albumin, a derivative of human blood with an extremely remote risk for viral diseases and Creutzfeldt-Jakob Disease. Less than 0.1% of patients receiving Hylenex have allergic reactions, however, anaphylactic-like reactions after Retrobulbar block or intravenous injections rarely have happened though most just have mild erythema and pain. Essentially, the On-Label use is only to enhance reactions with co-administered drugs.

Aesthetic Uses

Again, note that aesthetic and emergency applications to prevent or minimize necrosis or embolization after accidentally injecting blood vessels are Off-Label, as well as enzyme to sculpt HA fillers for smoothness and symmetry. This clearly must be part of any written informed consent, which should be integral to any hyaluronic acid filler consent authorizing emergency care automatically. Hyaluronic acid cosmetic injectable fillers cause catastrophic results when accidentally injected into blood vessels causing occlusion or embolization, resulting in skin necrosis, stroke, and – rarely – irreversible blindness.[48, 56] Consequently, our recommendation is to use blunt tip microcannula, particularly in areas which are considered higher risk.

Which Hyaluronidase?

So…which hyaluronidase should we use? Silverstein et al[57] compared the following different formulations in 2012 by their hyaluronidase activity per milligram total protein (U/mg)c:

1. recombinent human hyaluronidase—Hylenex 120,000
2. animal derived hyaluronidase 18,000
3. compounded animal derived hyaluronidase ~650

As you can see, the laboratory recombinent formulation, Hylenex, had far greater enzyme activity at 120,000 than the laboratory animal derived hyaluronidase at only 18,000. Trailing far behind, were five different individual compounding pharmacies which could average no more than 500 to 650 (U/mg)c with their less efficient processing equipment.

Most important, Hylenex, being non-animal derived, is the only formulation that does not require a preceding allergy skin test. In a true aesthetic medicine emergency there is no time to do skin allergy testing and certainly, we only want to use the most effective form of hyaluronidase. Consequently, in our practice, we only use Hylenex.[47]

How Much Time Do I Have?

The next consideration is to know how important it is to act quickly to dissolve hyaluronic acid filler when accidentally injected into a blood vessel. Kim et al[59] injected Restylane into the posterior auricular artery of rabbits then reversed the obstruction sequentially with hyaluronidase 4 hours and 24 hours later, comparing the zone of necrosis with each delay.

Tx 750 IU Hyaluronidase (Hyunidase) After 4 Hours or 24 Hours
Skin Necrosis After Enzyme at 4 hours...........0.04 cm^2
Skin Necrosis After Enzyme at 24 hours........10.10 cm^2

As expected, the zone of necrosis was much larger with the longer delay in reversing obstruction to blood flow. Consequently, the shorter the vascular obstruction time, the smaller the zone of necrosis, so speed is of the essence in this true aesthetic medicine emergency.

Which Areas Are Highest Risk for Blindness?

Jean & Alastair Carruthers, et al,[48, 58] tabulated the highest risk areas for the incidence of blindness from the accidental injection of cosmetic fillers in their definitive book: *Soft Tissue Augmentation*, in 2018, overlaying a face with symbols which reflect the frequency of occurrence in each high risk area. We highly recommend their reference to all cosmetic filler injectors, and their data is recreated below with our own model and graphics.

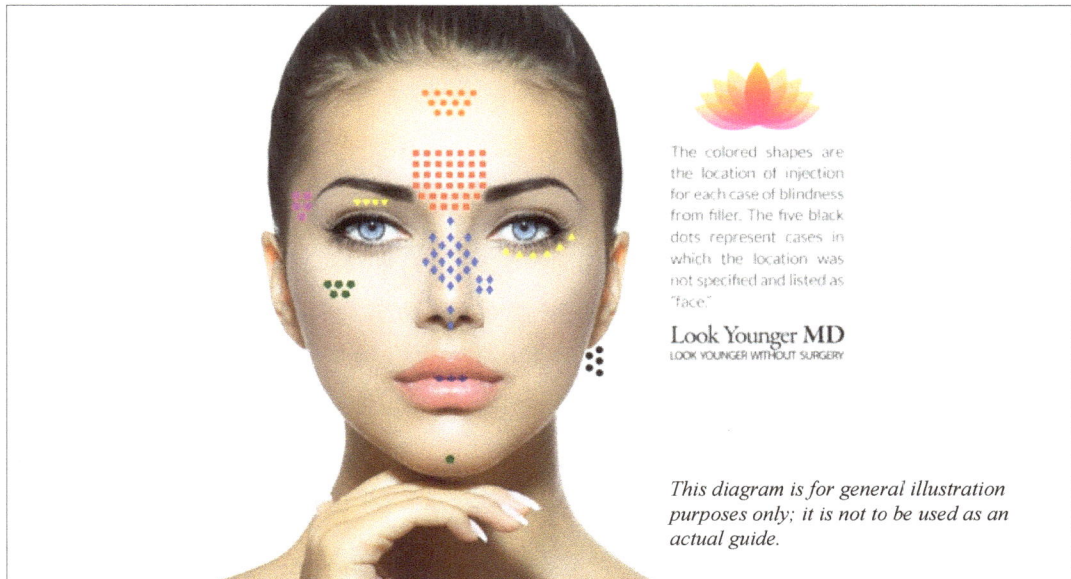

The colored shapes are the location of injection for each case of blindness from filler. The five black dots represent cases in which the location was not specified and listed as "face."

Look Younger MD
LOOK YOUNGER WITHOUT SURGERY

This diagram is for general illustration purposes only; it is not to be used as an actual guide.

You will note that the highest risk areas are the glabella between the eyes and the nose, and while other areas are indicated, no area with any blood flow can be considered completely safe. Despite our success injecting cosmetic filler in noses, we now refer nose corrections for surgery due to the heightened risk. Refer to Glabella Technique for our own current protocol as well as a summary of Jean and Alastair Caruthers latest glabella[3] technique published in 2018.

Emergency Cannulation Protocols

Emergency Standard of Care

We believe it is now the standard of care in 2019 for all cosmetic HA filler injectors to have an emergency protocol for reversal if there is an accidental HA injection into a blood vessel to prevent or minimize prolonged occlusion or embolization. Again, please note that our own protocols are not the Standard of Care – as none have been established yet – nevertheless, each injector can use the protocols presented as information upon which to construct your own Emergency Protocol.

Signs and Symptoms of Vascular Occlusion

This is characterized by the following signs or symptoms: momentary blanching leading to inflammation and erythema – particularly in a vascular pattern; painless to painful transition; swelling and dilatation of blood vessels; then ultimately, necrosis and/or CNS symptoms with embolization leading to stroke or blindness.[56, 57, 59] A classic finding[61, 64] is livedo reticularis (for a few days), a mottled reticulated vascular pattern with a lace-like purplish discoloration of the skin from swelling of the venules from obstruction of capillaries by small clots. This is often followed by blisters in about 3 days, then frank necrosis by day 6 unless properly treated.

DeLorenzi Vascular Occlusion (Non-Ocular) Enzyme Protocol

Claudio DeLorenzi,[61] MD, FRCS, a plastic surgeon in Ontario, Canada, initially proposed a protocol with one single daily treatment of hyaluronidase plus Nitropaste and hyperbaric oxygen, but ultimately found high doses of hyaluronidase repeated hourly (plus one baby aspirin a day for seven days) to be superior.

In 2017, he published the "New High Dosed Pulsed Hyaluronidase (HDPH) Protocol for Hyaluronic Acid Filler Vascular Adverse Events" in the Aesthetic Surgery Journal.[59] His protocol is to inject from 500 IU to 1,500 IU of hyaluronidase every hour depending upon the apparent surface area affected – determined by delayed capillary refill in the area affected. His "HYAL Flooding Hypothesis" is that HA filler obstructed arteries need to be bathed in high concentrations of hyaluronidase for long periods of time to dissolve the filler.

He uses only the number of ischemic surface areas to estimate the tissue volume of the affected underlying area to compute his doses. For example, each hour, he uses 500 IU for half of the right upper lip (to the NL fold), but uses 1,000 IU when the right upper lip extends to the nose. He also uses 500 IU hourly in the entire glabella area; and he uses 1,500 IU hourly for half of the right ML, right NL, and nose areas.

Interestingly, he no longer uses any of the other proposed ancillary treatments like Nitropaste and hyperbaric oxygen, deeming them as unnecessary in view of the dominant success of his protocol. The only exception is the daily use of a baby aspirin for a week which he believes useful to reduce platelet activity.

He recommends using compression of the skin with an instrument and comparing the capillary refill with that of adjacent tissue – or tissue on the opposing side of the face as a control. We suggest if no such instrument is available, that the tip of a straw may be used to estimate this. Moreover, as the enzyme works, fragments of the dissolved filler may travel downstream to cause micro-infarcts or injuries and a delayed effect of the original obstruction. The ideal interval of hyaluronidase treatment has yet to be determined, so his hourly protocol may ultimately be found to be excessive, but clinical trials will be necessary.

Retrobulbar Injection

Recently, there have been rare case reports of the reversal of the temporary blindness from cosmetic filler injections using the Retrobulbar[60, 61, 64] injection technique for hyaluronidase, though the success rates are low and the risks and inherent difficulty of injection during a medical emergency are considerable. Conceivably, one could go blind just from inexperience with the injection procedure itself, and given that the window of time for treatment of the central retinal artery is no more than ~90 minutes[48] – this is almost impossible in the referral and transport time necessary – unless it can be done on-site where the inadvertent injection occurred.

Ocular Vascular Occlusion Retrobulbar[60, 61, 64] Enzyme Protocol

Heretofore, we have described successful protocols after accidental injection of HA fillers into facial blood vessels resulting in localized effects to skin and soft tissue with profound success in reversal using 2019 enzyme protocols.

We have not described what can be done if injectable filler embolization results in distal and central affects like stroke or occlusion of the retinal artery leading to vision loss. This is a rare occurrence, so little more than anecdotal reports have surfaced with few reports of success using the Retrobulbar injection technique.[62, 63]

In summary, a Retrobulbar needle (25 or 27 gauge, 1.5 inch) is inserted through the skin at the junction of the lateral 1/3 and medical 2/3s of the infraorbital rim. The patient is directed to look superior and medial and the needle is advanced 1 to 2 cm along the bottom of the orbit. After crossing the mid-point of the globe, the needle is then directed medially and superiorly toward the apex of the orbit. Once there is a negative blood aspiration, 1,500 IU or 3,000 IU of hyaluronidase is injected.

As you can deduce, aside from the low rate of success in restoration of vision, this is a daunting task for anyone not versed in the process of doing Retrobulbar injections, particularly as the procedure itself can result in blindness. Consequently, our plan is to use the following approach:

Ocular Vascular Occlusion – Supraorbital[34] Notch Enzyme Protocol

In 2015 a highly experienced aesthetic nurse inadvertently injected a patient in Australia who immediately complained of vision loss after injection of HA filler. Fortunately, Mike Clague,[34] BSC, had the brilliant inspiration to inject hyaluronidase directly and repeatedly directly into the supratrochlear and supraorbital notch. He bathed the patient with direct injections of more than 600 IU of hyaluronidase and kept doing this until the patient had complete visual acuity resolution.

The supraorbital notch and the supratrochlear have the incredible advantage of being far more accessible in an emergency than the Retrobulbar eye injection approach, have far less inherent risk from the injection itself, and could possibly be done by cosmetic injectors who are not experienced eye surgeons. In our own protocol, we focus only upon the supraorbital to minimize potential damage to ocular muscles and stipulate a 27 gauge 1" needle. We recommend transport immediately to the local hospital and with ocular specialty referral and consideration for hyperbaric oxygen treatments.

I had the distinct pleasure to hear Michael Clague, BSC, and Dermatologist Ava Shamban present in person in Santa Monica, CA, in February 2019, and highly recommend their lecture program (www.facecoachlive.com) to any who wish to become an expert at cosmetic injectable fillers.

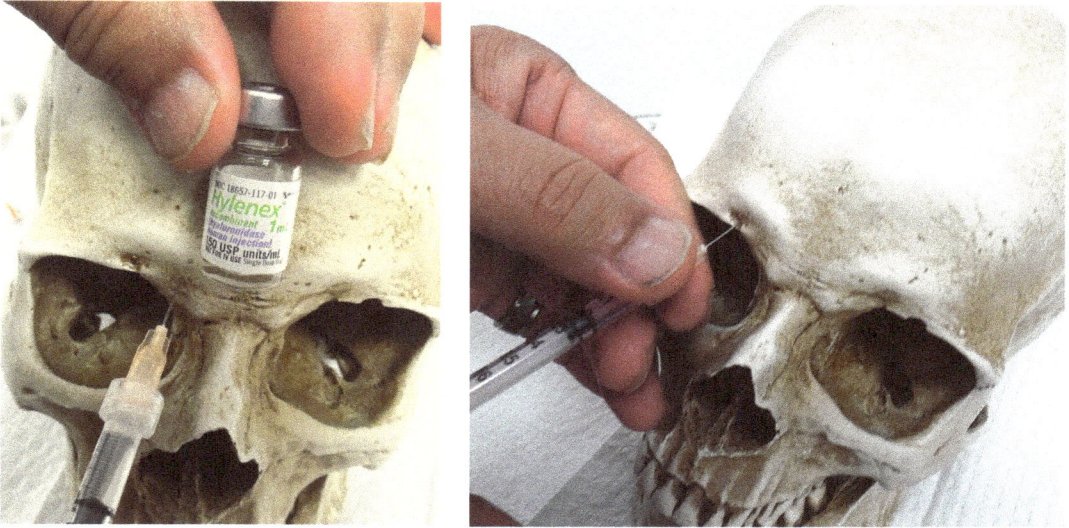

A drawback of high dose hyaluronidase injections is that the typical clinic usually cannot afford to have enough enzyme on hand since the cost for Hylenex, the only form that does not require skin allergy testing, is at the time of this writing $78/cc per 150 IU bottle, with an expiration date of only a few months. Consequently, four bottles are only a starter dose, so I recommend several practices in an area agree beforehand to pool their Hylenex as a reserve for immediate purchase by any single practice in an ocular emergency.

Email us at **LookYoungerMD@gmail.com** if you would like us to connect you with other clinics in your immediate area to inquire if this is possible. If we receive more than one inquiry in a particular city, we will forward your interest to each of you to determine if you can make this possible.

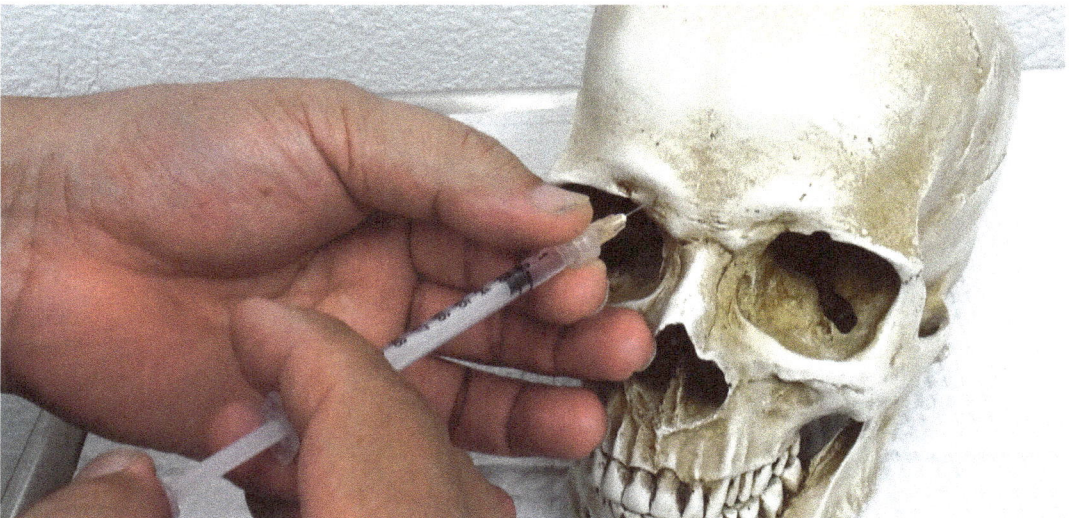

Before/After Immediate Injection of Hylenex Into Right Temple
for Cannulation of Vein After Juvederm® Injection

Remember that hyaluronidase enzyme is only truly effective with hyaluronic acid cosmetic injectable fillers, such as Juvederm,® Restylane,® and Belotero Balance,® which is a primary consideration in my selection of them as cosmetic injectable fillers. Consequently, it is unknown if hyaluronidase has any affect at all upon non-HA cosmetic injectable fillers.

Enzyme Sculpting

Non-Emergency Use of Hyaluronidase to Sculpt Filler

Off-Label, we also used hyaluronidase aesthetically to sculpt HA cosmetic injectable fillers for smoothness and symmetry.[1, 43]

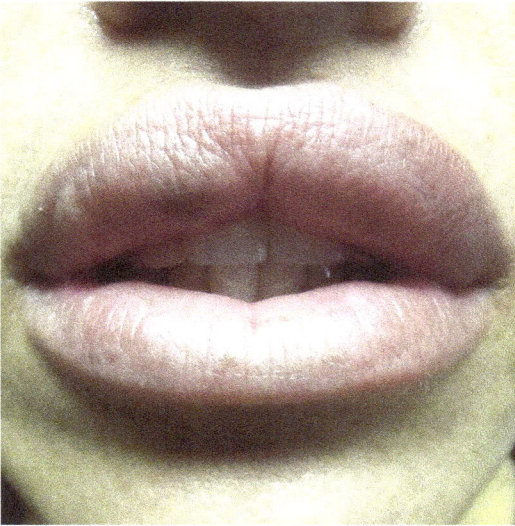

Excessive Upper Lip HA Filler

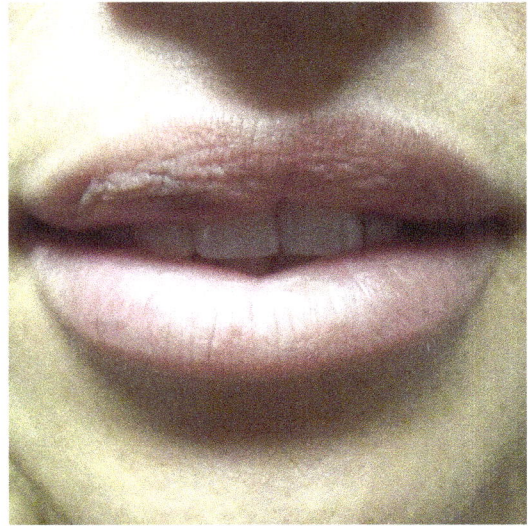

Partial Correction After Hylenex Injection

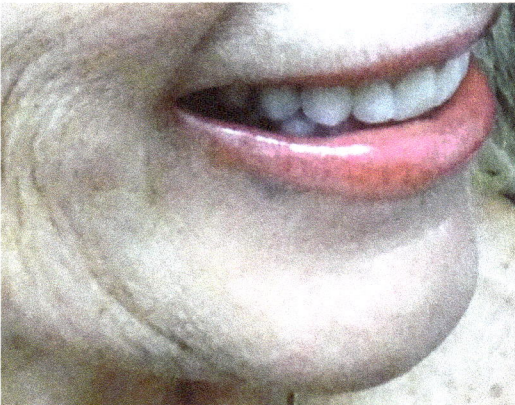

Blue Tyndall Effect Right Lower Lip

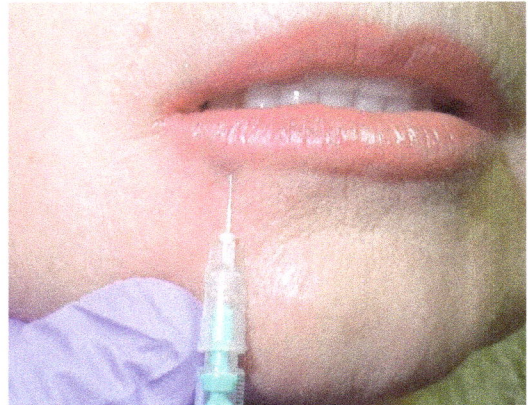

Correction of Tyndall with Hylenex

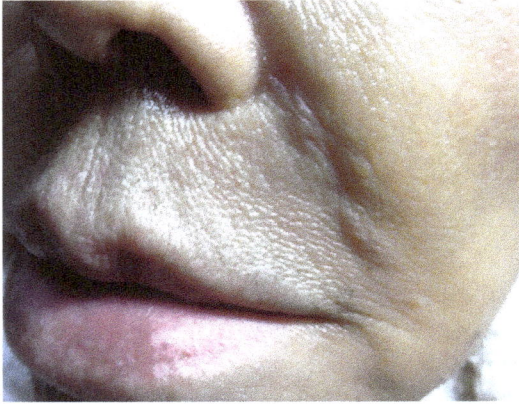

Superficial HA Injection Into NL Folds

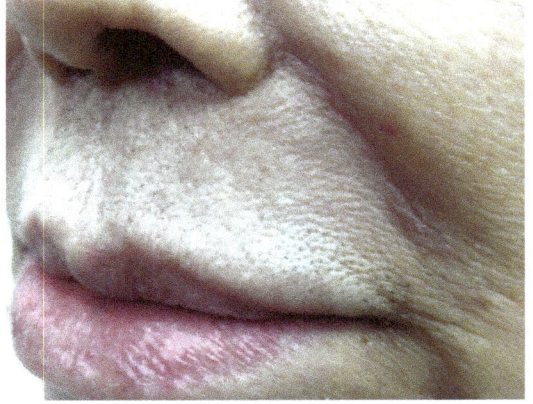

Correction with Hylenex Injections

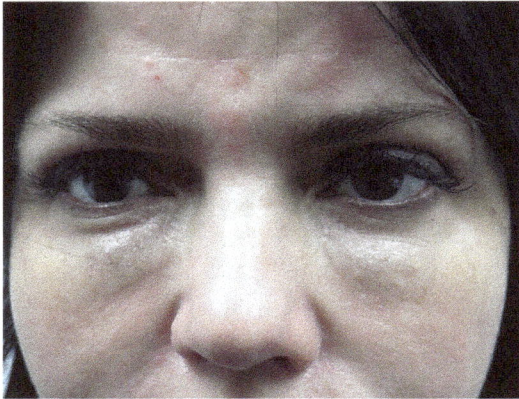

Mid-Cheek Overfill with HA Filler

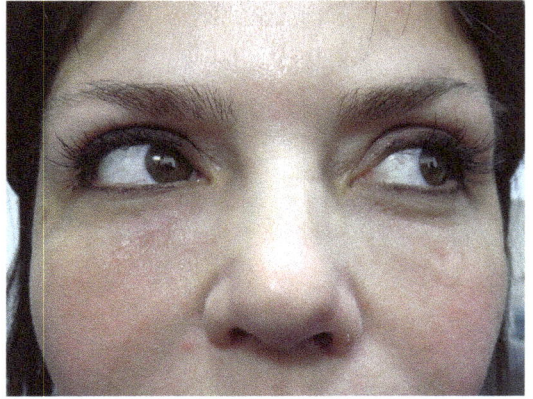

Mid-Cheek After Hylenex Correction

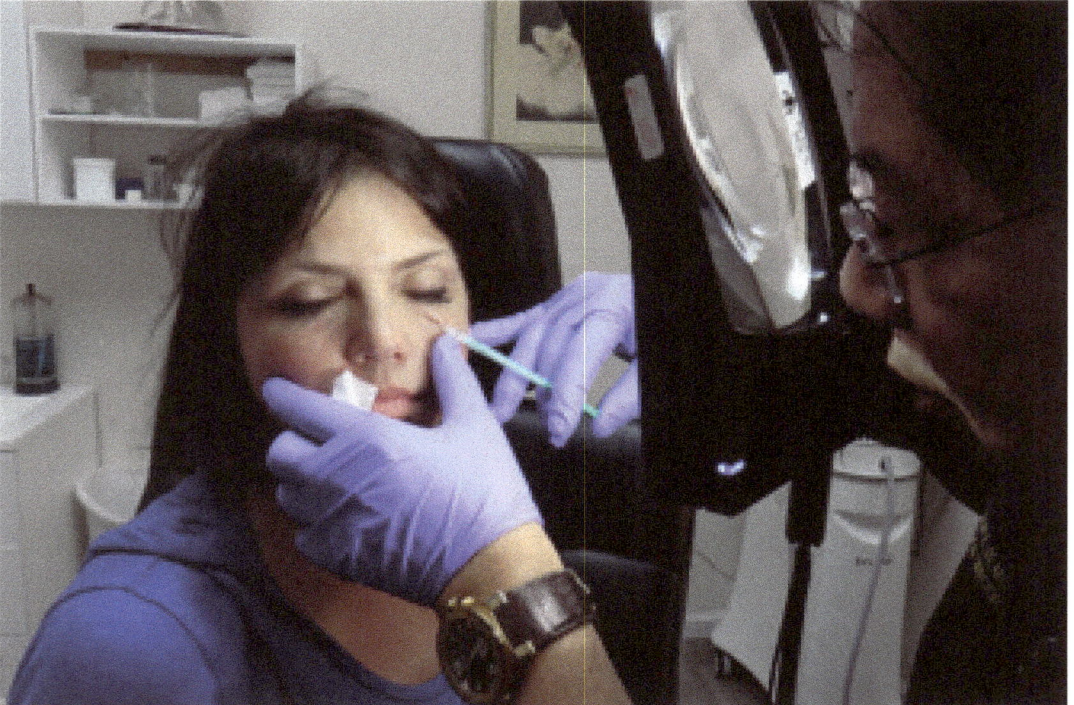

Our protocol is to initially draw up 0.10 cc (15 IU) into a one cc syringe and to inject directly into any excessive areas of HA filler with a 32 gauge ½" needle, followed by gentle massage focused mostly at bringing the enzyme and excessive HA product directly into contact with each other. We then wait 3 to 5 minutes because there is usually an immediate result, and repeat at 5 minute intervals at 15 to 30 IU as needed if only partially successful. Remarkably, the enzyme has the ability to penetrate blood vessels if in proximity, but of course is most effective if the enzyme is injected as directly as possible into the cosmetic filler.

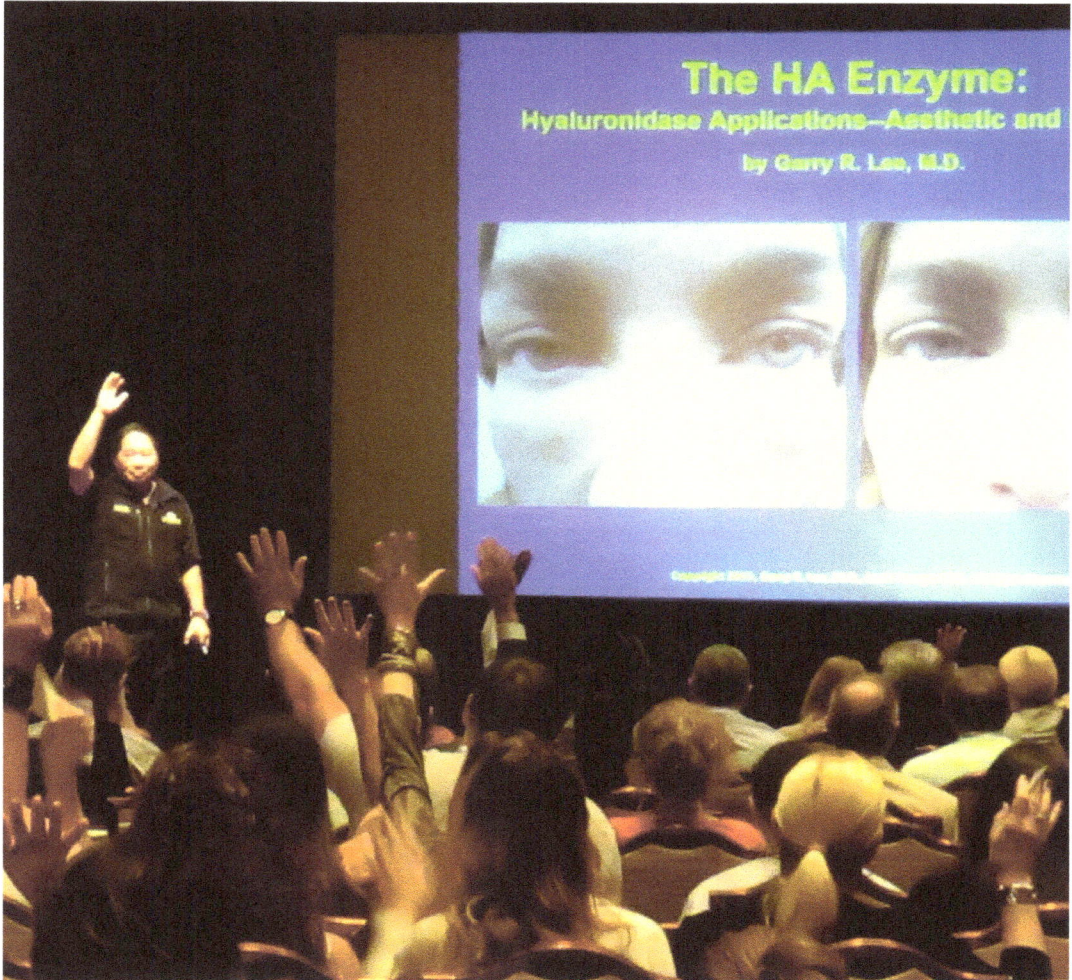

Dr. Lee Lecturing to Physicians on Off-Label
Hyaluronidase Enzyme Aesthetic & Emergent Treatments

NOTES

Anti-Pain and Anti-Bruising Protocols

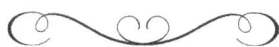

Blunt Tip, Ice, and Topical Numbing

Of course the microcannula itself, by virtue of its blunt tip, is inherently less painful and with the application of the Wiggle Progression Technique, appears to cause less bruising because it is less likely to penetrate blood vessels.

Fortunately, for most patients, topical compounded numbing cream together with the topical application of ice is adequate for more than 95% of our cosmetic injection patients. Our protocol is simply to use BLT applied topically for 10 minutes on the areas to be treated on the face. If we are applying BLT to a significant surface area of the body, lidocaine toxicity must be considered, though the application simply to the buttocks – our largest area – is such a small area as to be of no concern.

We also briefly apply topical ice just before and after each injection to minimize discomfort and to minimize bleeding. If bleeding is not readily controlled, direct pressure works after a few minutes unless there is a coagulation issue.

Nevertheless, it is useful to have a greater ability to diminish pain and anxiety for those who may have need of it. The problem is that outpatient pain control for the most powerful skin rejuvenation, laser tattoo removal, and skin tightening procedures often uses a combination of anxiolytic medications such as Xanax® or Halcion;® a narcotic, such as Lortab® or Percocet;® topical numbing agents; nerve blocks such as the Inferior Orbital Nerve and Mental Nerve; and local lidocaine injections into treatment areas.

This is inconvenient as oral pain and anxiety medications often lead to patient impairment, increasing liability as well as requiring someone else to drive the patient to and from treatment. On the other hand, injections can be time consuming, incorporating a number of hypodermic needle injections with concomitant pain, bruising, and swelling.

In our first book, we recommended Microcannula Injected Local Anesthesia (MILA), the use of aesthetic microcannula to inject local anesthesia instead of the conventional use for the injection of cosmetic wrinkle fillers. However we discontinued MILA when we found it to be slower to inject than the conventional use of hypodermic needles with only a marginal decrease in the apparent pain.

PRO-NOX™ (nitrous oxide)

In 2019, we now use the PRO-NOX™[66] nitrous oxide device – commonly known as laughing gas – for those whose mild pain[66, 67] cannot be adequately controlled with the application of ice and topical numbing cream, particularly when we combine our injections with energy devices. It has the advantage of reducing anxiety as well as fairly significant pain control, which in most cases is sufficient for those with needle phobia.

The cardinal advantages of PRO-NOX™ are that the administered concentration is strictly limited to 50% of nitrous oxide and 50% O_2, obviating the need for an anesthesiologist for administration; that it is by self-inhalation; and that

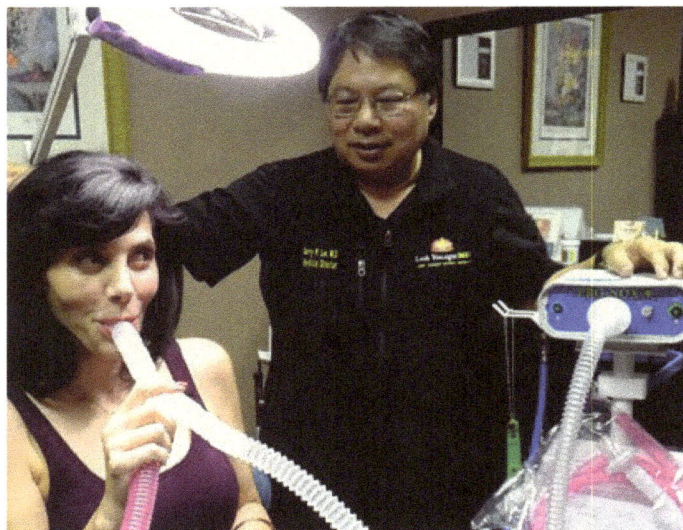

it is so rapidly cleared by respiration that patients may drive home just minutes after treatment. Of course, traditional dentistry has used nitrous oxide for years, particularly with pediatric patients, but it was not until PRO-NOX™ designed a minimal risk system that we found the pharmaceutical regulatory controls and the concurrent risk reduction to be minimal enough, at an acceptable price, for application to minimally invasive aesthetic medicine. In modern day aesthetic medicine, our ability to produce results with minimal overhead costs and greater patient convenience creates the value essential to success.

AccuVein™ Navigation & Mapping

Fortunately, we now have the advantage of laser technology to help us more precisely place blood vessels to approximately 1 cm in depth using the AccuVein™ [29] System. AccuVein™ uses 2 lasers to isolate the hemoglobin within blood vessels to painlessly visualize their location beneath the skin which we use to help us avoid vasculature hazards – the land mines, if you will – of cosmetic filler injection.

Predominately used for venipuncture in major laboratories, I first saw the aesthetic application by JD McCoy, MD, where he actively used the AccuVein™ in real time as he injected Sculptra® into the buttocks as a contouring agent to shape them more attractively. AccuVein™ has a custom designed device holder

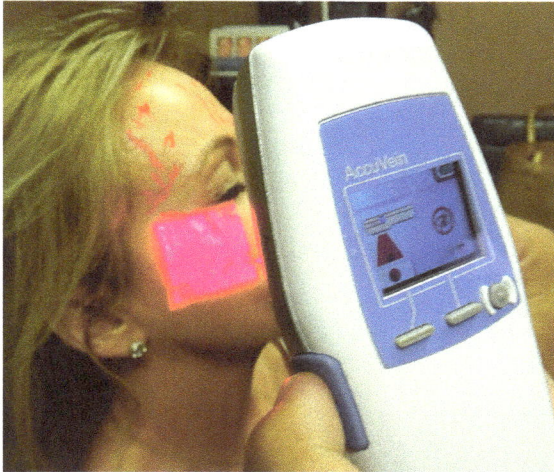

which may be purchased additionally, which is quite effective to adjust and to project the laser over a particular area, however, particularly in the face, I find the use of the AccuVein™ to interfere with the depth perception I need to determine the sequential placement of cosmetic injectable filler. AccuVein™ can be used in normal ambient indoor lighting, but high intensity light tends to wash out the visibility of detail.

Consequently, we have shifted from using the AccuVein™ in real time to simply using a surgical marker to outline the major blood vessels in the treatment area. I find the AccuVein™ to be highly effective in helping us to avoid most large and superficial blood vessels, but its effectiveness is limited to only about a depth of 1.0 cm – missing critical deeper blood vessels – as well as, in our case, by the amount and accuracy of surgical marking our staff uses in clinical preparation.

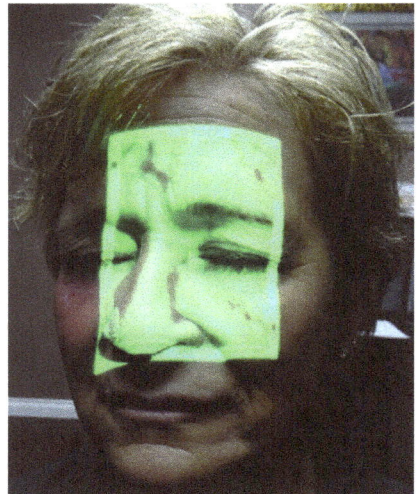

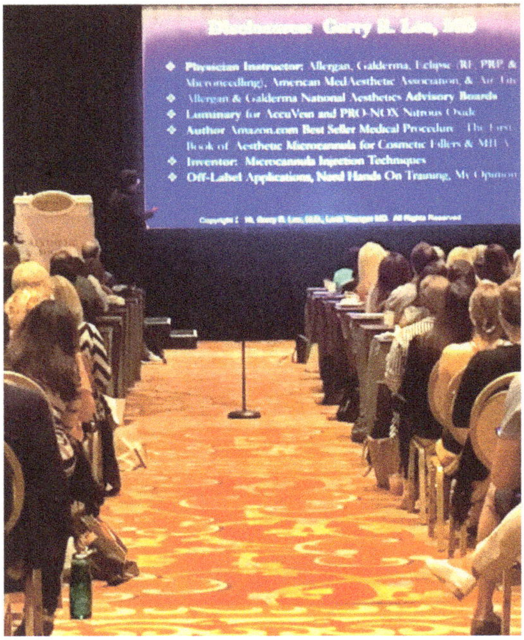

NOTES

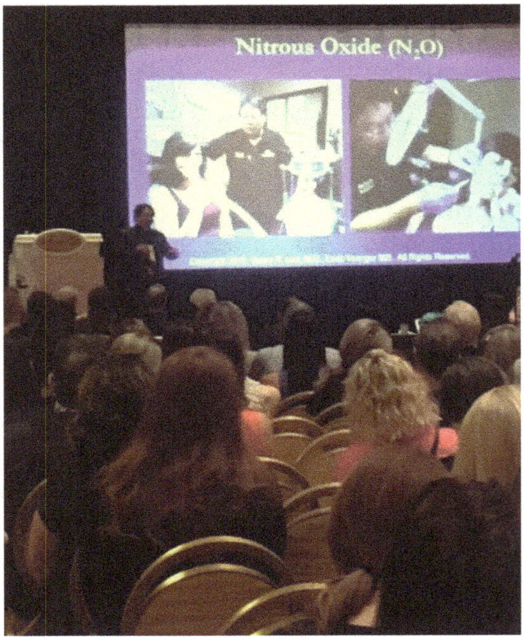

_____

_____

_____

_____

_____

_____

_____

_____

_____

_____

_____

_____

_____

_____

Using Microcannula to Dissolve Sculptra® Nodules

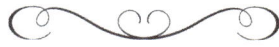

Instead of repeatedly injecting a patient over and over again with a hypodermic needle, microcannula can also be used to dissolve Sculptra® nodules using a 27 gauge 1½" TSK STERiGLIDE microcannula. The Pilot hole is made adjacent to the nodule and 1-2 cc of Lidocaine is injected to dissolve the accumulation. When absorbed, the nodule becomes malleable and the tip of the microcannula can be repeatedly injected in a Basic Fan pattern to break up the nodule. Typically, several sessions are required for complete resolution, depending upon the size and age of the Sculptra® nodule.

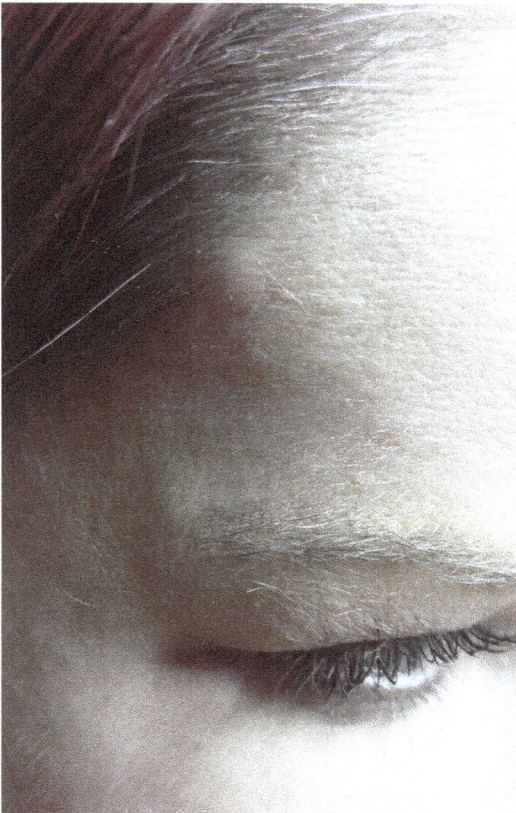

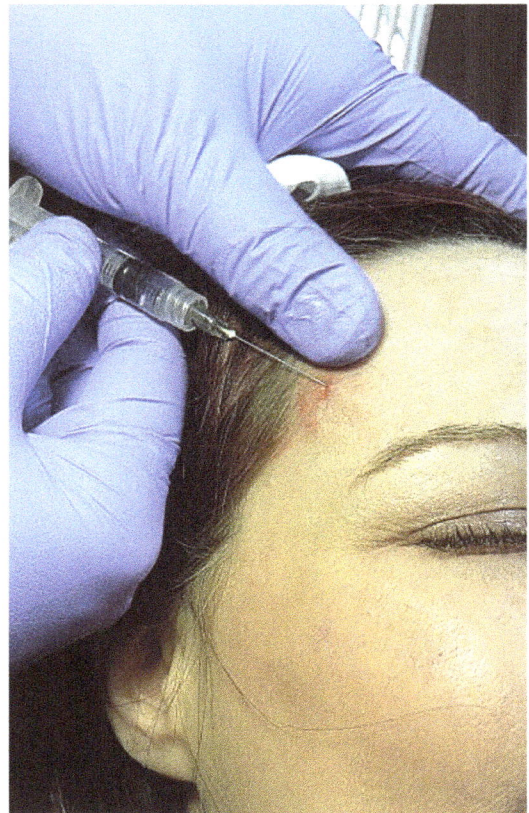

Right Temple Sculptra® Nodule from Inadequate Massage
Injected with Lidocaine Using Microcannula

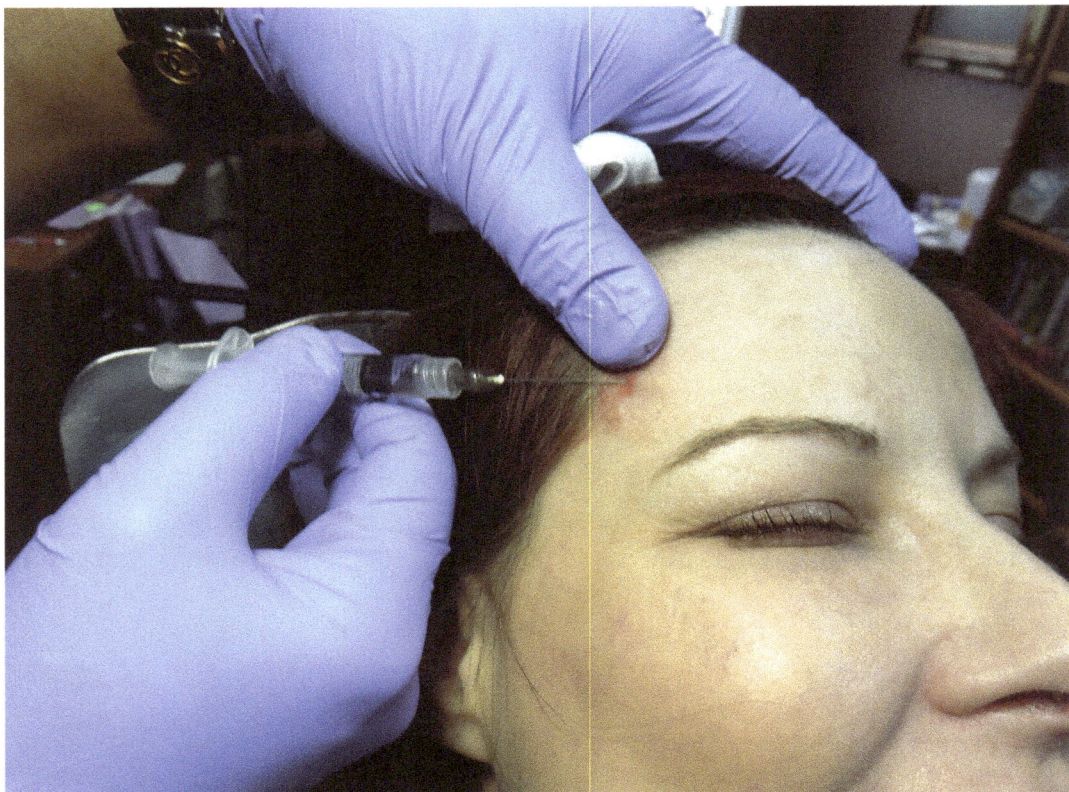

Injection of Lidocaine Into Nodule Using the Microcannula Fanning Technique

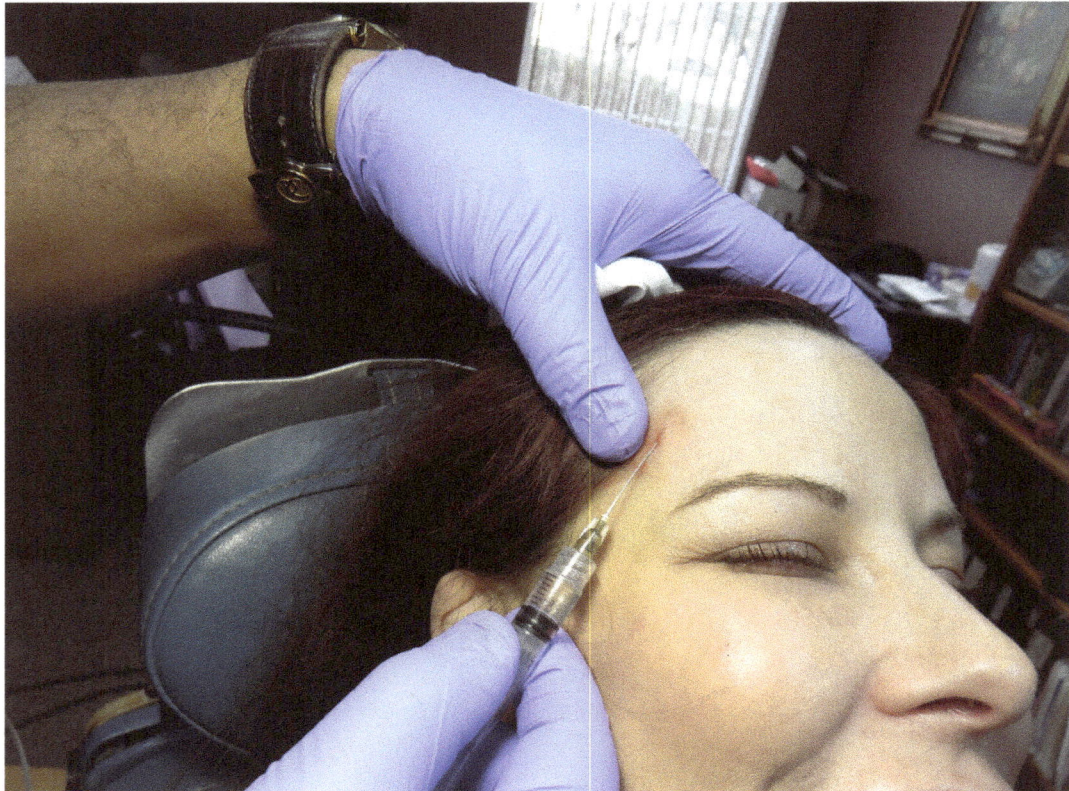

Future Trends

Finally…the Great American Recession has given way to an economy – so unexpectedly strong – that the concern is in reining it in so that inflation does not become the presenting issue. In 2019, this has driven the reemergence of interest to do cosmetic procedures, particularly non-invasive ones which tend to be less costly procedurally and with minimal down time.

The American Society for Aesthetic Plastic Surgery[23] recorded that soft tissue HA fillers increased 12.2% from 2017 to 2018; and 58.4% from 2014 to 2018. After Botulinum toxin, it is the most utilized minimally-invasive cosmetic procedure in the USA, with hyaluronic acid filler use clearly dominating at an astounding 93.1% of all injectable fillers for 2018 (810,240 of a total of 870,097 procedures). Further, since the US market penetration for cosmetic injectable fillers is estimated to be only at 6% of its ultimate potential[68] in 2019, the immediate future of this industry is bright, indeed.

In aesthetic medicine, we often the get the best cosmetic results with Plastic Surgery – our most painful and expensive interventional procedures – which correspondingly require the longest recovery time. Consequently, many patients tend to avoid surgery if they seek less painful treatments with less recovery time – as well as for its inherent risks and the associated costs of an anesthesiologist and a hospital or a surgical center. Hence, for these patients, the solution they seek is in the best cosmetic results we can accomplish safely and comfortably in an outpatient setting.

When I first lectured on the use of microcannula in place of hypodermic needles in 2012, I spoke of the "revolution" I predicted this would bring to our industry. Subsequent to this, I described the continuous growth as an "evolution" in our techniques. Today, I characterize where we are as an increasing "convolution" of minimally invasive technologies working in concert together towards achieving the best possible results.

We are now commonly using Platelet-Rich Plasma (PRP) in aesthetics though the only USA FDA indication to date is for orthopedic surgery and aesthetic benefits to date are more anecdotal than evidence based. On the horizon, I believe that the next frontier in minimally invasive cosmetic medicine will be in the combination of microcannula introduced cosmetic fillers with synergistic modalities – such as laser, radio frequency, microneedling, stem cells, and PRP.

The challenge today is how to best integrate these together. What we are seeing is a convergence of technologies in which our incremental advances in outpatient non-invasive cosmetic medicine treatment and local anesthesia may one day produce results which begin to rival – what we can only see today – with plastic surgery.

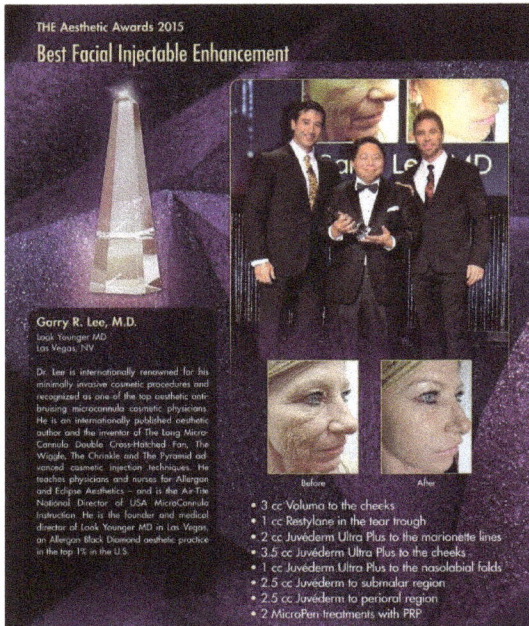

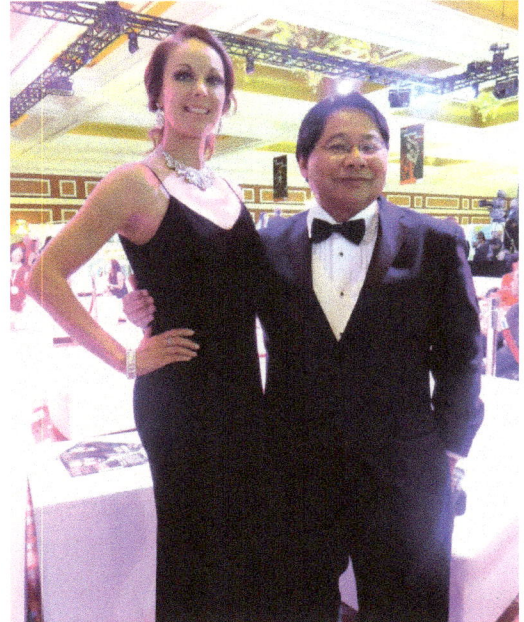

WINNER of The Aesthetic Award 2015 for Best Facial Injectable Enhancement in the USA

About The Author

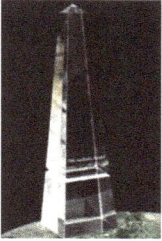

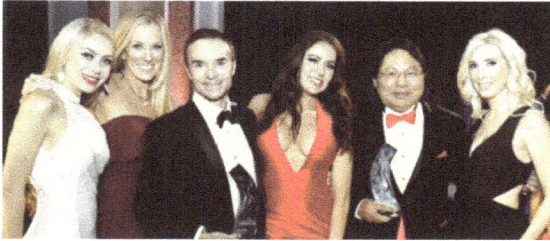

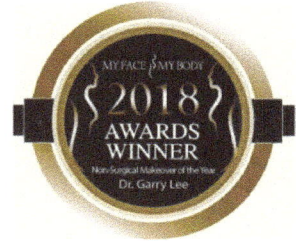

Dr. Lee is the USA's Triple Crown Award WINNER to help you "Look Younger, Without Surgery," internationally selected as one of the Ultimate 100 Global Aesthetic Leaders in the World in 2019 by MyFaceMyBody, the World's Largest and Most Recognized Awards Program.

He is the National Winner of the Top 3 Cosmetic Injection Awards in the United States: 1) The Aesthetic Award as *The Best Facial Injectable Enhancement Physician* in the USA in 2015– endorsed by Plastic Surgeon Andrew Ordon of TV's "The Doctors," 2) *The Top Aesthetic Doctor* in the USA for the Aesthetic Everything 2019 Aesthetic and Cosmetic Medicine Awards, 3) and *The Best Non-Surgical Makeover* in the USA in 2018 for MyFaceMyBody, selected by an International Panel of Judges, including Plastic Surgeon Paul Nassif, of TV's "Botched," in competition with hundreds of the Top Plastic Surgeons and Dermatologists in the USA.

He also led the USA to take Second Place in WORLD Competition for the *Best Non-Surgical Facial Rejuvenation* among 31 of the Top Physicians from 5 Continents at the Aesthetic & Anti-Aging Medicine European Congress (AMEC) in Paris, France.

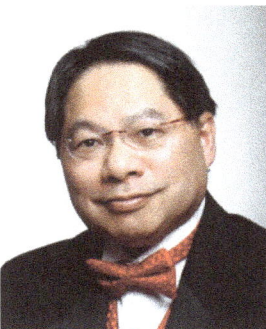

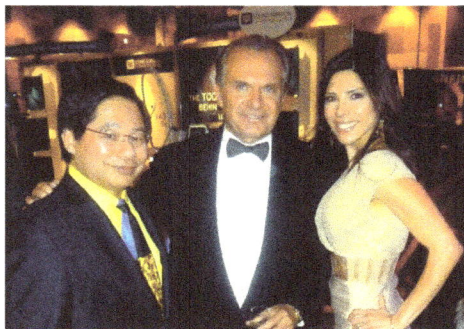

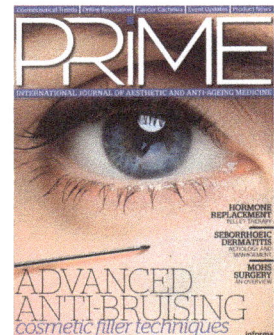

Dr. Lee served on the Allergan (Botox®/Juvederm®) Medical Facial Aesthetics USA Advisory Board, the Allergan New Core Advisory Board, and the Galderma (Dysport®/Restylane®) National Advisory Board. He lectured for The Aesthetic Show, The American Society of Cosmetic Physicians, The American Academy of Anti-Aging Medicine, Vegas Cosmetic Surgery & Aesthetic Dermatology, The Canadian Association of Aesthetic Medicine, and The American MedAesthetic Association. He instructed physicians and nurses for Allergan (Botox® and Juvederm®), Galderma (Dysport® and Restylane®), Eclipse (microneedling, PRP, & RF), and – most recently – the Cellular Medicine Association (O-Shot, Vampire Face Lift), and is the Air-Tite National Director of USA MicroCannula Physician Instruction.

Dr. Lee is the Author of the *First Book of Aesthetic Microcannula for Cosmetic Fillers & Local Anesthesia,* Amazon.com's 2016 Best Seller for Medical Procedure. He is an internationally published author in peer-reviewed *PRiME: International Journal of Aesthetic & Anti-Ageing Medicine* and his articles, case photos, and opinions are repeatedly published in *MedEsthetics* and *The Aesthetic Guide Magazines* for plastic surgeons and dermatologists throughout the USA. Dr. Lee and Plastic Surgeon Gordon Sasaki co-authored an article on Platelet-Rich Plasma (PRP) in the treatment of androgenetic alopecia in the September 2014 issue of *MedEsthetics Magazine.*

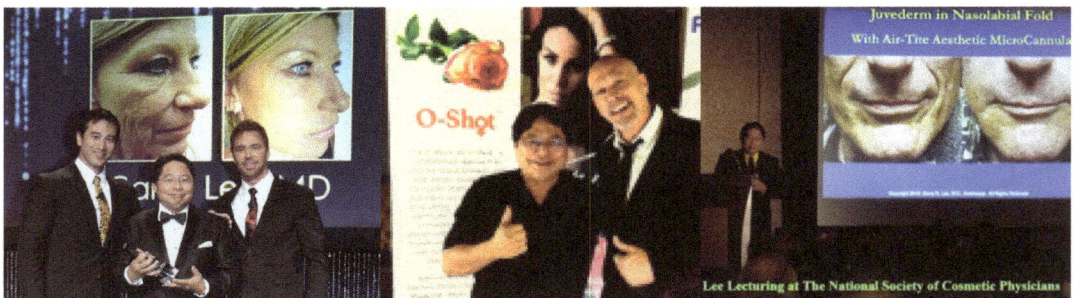

Lee Lecturing at The National Society of Cosmetic Physicians

CME/CEU Training:
Webinar & Hands-On

We invite you to join us for CME and CEU training conducted at the National Award WINNING level…directly from Dr. Lee. Click the link at **LookYoungerMd.com** for high quality continuing education credit specifically for minimally invasive cosmetic medicine. On a limited and selective basis, Dr. Lee teaches personal onsite Workshops and Preceptorships at his clinic, Look Younger MD, in Las Vegas, Nevada. Feel free to just call us at 702-938-0190 or email us at LookYoungerMD@gmail.com with any questions.

If you are unable to join us, use the following criteria to select the highest quality CME and CEU instruction in your local area:

So…how do you tell a mediocre CME & CEU instructor…from someone GREAT?

Continuing Medical Education (CME/CEU/CE) accreditation is primarily concerned with having the appropriate Board Certification as the minimal basis for competence and avoiding brand bias – but the ability to do minimally invasive aesthetic medicine and the ability to teach varies tremendously by the experience and individual skill of each physician.

For example – having Board Certification in Plastic Surgery – is no guarantee that your Instructor will be GREAT. The very best Plastic Surgeons often spend most of their time in surgery and delegate their non-surgical cosmetic treatments to their assistants. Consequently, their nurse or PA – who does it full-time – may actually be better than the Board Certified Plastic Surgeon who only does it part-time.

We were astounded so many Continuing Medical Education programs were charging unsuspecting doctors, nurses, and physician assistants anywhere up to $4,000 per attendee for CME & CEU training – with mediocre instructors.

To help you, Dr. Lee compiled the *Five (5) Steps To Find a **GREAT** Aesthetic*

Cosmetic Injection Instructor, beginning at the bottom (brown step) of the Credentialing Pyramid below:

Does YOUR Doctor Measure Up?

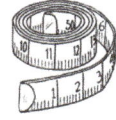

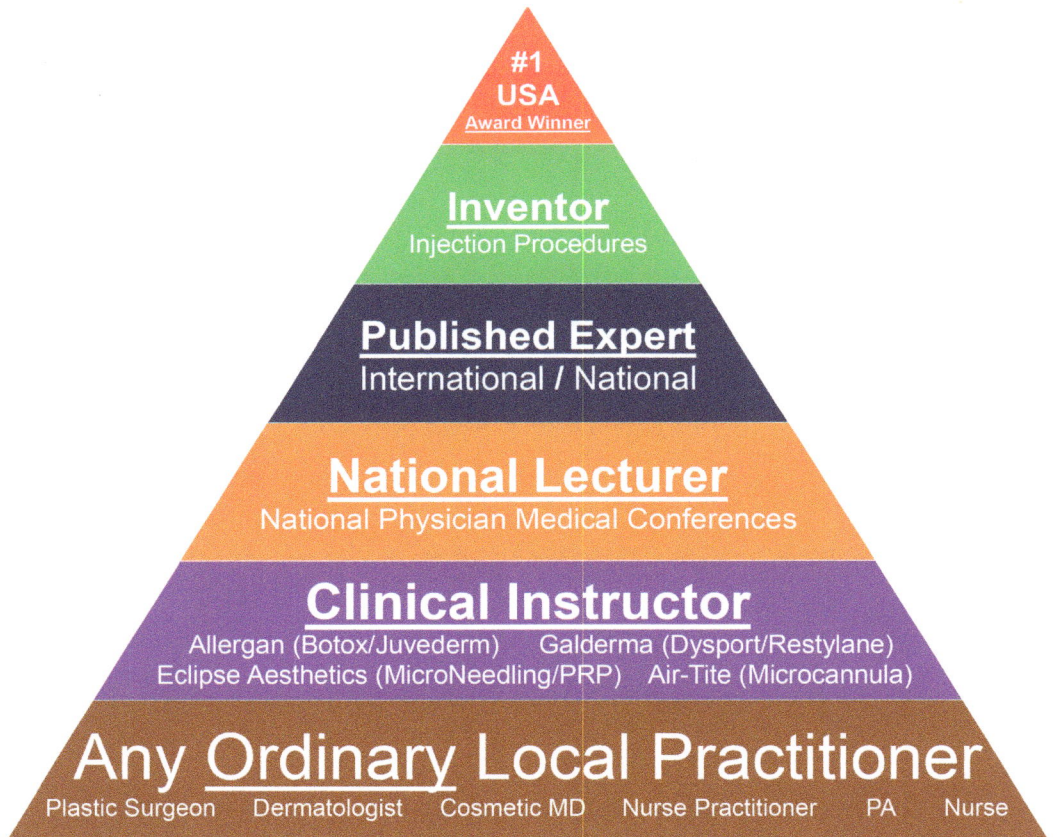

#1 USA Award Winner

Inventor
Injection Procedures

Published Expert
International / National

National Lecturer
National Physician Medical Conferences

Clinical Instructor
Allergan (Botox/Juvederm)   Galderma (Dysport/Restylane)
Eclipse Aesthetics (MicroNeedling/PRP)   Air-Tite (Microcannula)

Any Ordinary Local Practitioner
Plastic Surgeon   Dermatologist   Cosmetic MD   Nurse Practitioner   PA   Nurse

Garry R. Lee, MD—Selected One of the Ultimate 100 Global Aesthetic Leaders in the WORLD for 2019. The WINNER of the TOP Cosmetic Injection Awards in the USA…endorsed by Plastic Surgeon Andrew Ordon of TV's "The Doctors" and Judged by Plastic Surgeon Paul Nassif of TV's "Botched." Dr. Lee is the Inventor of Microcannula Cosmetic Injection Techniques, an Amazon.com Best Selling Author for Medical Procedure, a National Lecturer on Cosmetic Injections, and Clinical Instructor for Allergan (Botox/Juvederm), Galderma (Dysport/Restylane), Eclipse (PRP), SkinPen, Air-Tite (Microcannula) and the CMA (The O-Shot).

See LookYoungerMD.com

1. Dark Brown Level

Of the 700+ Allergan (Botox®/Juvederm®) and Galderma (Dysport®/Restylane®) accounts in the Las Vegas and the surrounding area, only the TOP 1% are selected to be <u>Clinical Instructors</u> to teach doctors and nurses.

2. Periwinkle Blue Level

Of the Clinical Instructors, only a few are hand-picked to be a <u>National Lecturer</u> to teach at physician medical conferences in the USA.

3. Light Brown Level

Of the National Lecturers, only a few are chosen by the Editors of National or International Journal to be a <u>Published Author</u> as an expert in the USA or the World.

4. Purple Level

Of the Published Authors, only a tiny fraction are <u>Inventors</u> whose products or techniques are used within the industry.

5. Green Level

Of the Inventors, only the Best of the Best compete and win <u>National Awards</u> in TOP competition from Beverly Hills to New York City, to Paris, and beyond.

6. Red Level

The #1 National and International Aesthetic Medicine <u>Award Winners</u>.

NOTES

References

1. Lee, Garry. The First Book of Aesthetic Microcannula For Cosmetic Fillers & Local Anesthesia (MILA) © 2016; IngramSpark

2. Stoelting, R. and Miller, R. Basics of Anesthesia, Fifth Edition, p. 5-6. Copyright © 2007 Churchill Livingstone an imprint of Elsevier Inc.

3. Carruthers, Jean, et al. Soft Tissue Augmentation. 4th ed., Elsevier, 2018; pg 17

4. Carruthers, Jean, et al. Soft Tissue Augmentation. 4th ed., Elsevier, 2018; pg 17-56, 97-99

5. Sherman, Richard, MD. Avoiding Dermal Filler Complications. Clinics In Dermatology. 2009; 27,s23-s32

6. Glogau R, and Kane M. Effect of Injection Techniques on the Rate of Local Adverse Events in Patients Implanted with Non-animal Hyaluronic Acid Gel Dermal Fillers. Dermatol Surg 2008; 34: S105– S109

7. Tzikas TL. Evaluation of the Radiance FN Soft tissue Filler for Facial Soft Tissue Augmentation. Arch Facial Plast Surg. 2004; 6(4): 234-239

8. Zeichner JA, Cohen JL. Use of Blunt Tip Cannulas for Soft Tissue Fillers. J Drugs Dermatol. 2012; 11(1): 70-72

9. Lee, G. Advanced Anti-Bruising Cosmetic Filler Techniques. PRiME International Journal of Aesthetic and Anti-Ageing Medicine. January/February 2015, Volume 5, Issue 1, p.25-34

10. Chesnut C., Hsiao J., Beynet D. New Uses for Fillers. Cosmetic Dermatology. 2012;25:176-182

11. Niamtu J., III. Filler Injection with Micro-Cannula Instead of Needles. Dermatol Surg. 2009; 35(12): 2005-2008

12. Niamtu, J., III. Novel Cannulas Impart Filler Treatments with Less Bruising, Downtime for Patients. Cosmetic Surgery Times. July 1, 2011

13. Merriam-Webster Online Dictionary and Thesaurus. Available at: http://www.merriam-webster.com/dictionary/cannula [Last assessed 21 June 2019]

14. Prosotu Cannula and Needle Solutions. Available at: http://prosotu. com/cannula-and-needles/ [Last assessed 21 June 2019]

15. Fulton J., Caperton C., Dewandre L. Filler Injections with the Blunt-tip Microcannula. Journal of Drugs in Dermatology. 2012; 11(9): 1098-103

16. Hexsel D., Soirefmann M., Porto MD., Siega C., Shcilling-Souza J., Brum C. Double-Blind, Randomized, Controlled Clinical Trial to Compare

Safety and Efficacy of a Metallic Cannula with that of a Standard Needle for Soft Tissue Augmentation of the Nasolabial Folds. Dermatologic Surgery. 2012; 38(2): 207-14

17. Lazzeri D., Agostini T., Figus M., Nardi M., Pantaloni M. Lazzeri S. Blindness Following Cosmetic Injections of the Face. Plast. Reconstr. Surg. 2012; 129: 995

18. Hamman M., Goldman M. Minimizing Bruising Following Fillers and Other Cosmetic Injectables. J Clin Aesthet Dermatol Aug 2013; 6(8):16-18

19. Lee, G. Physician Instructor Discusses Advantages of Microcannulas for Dermal Filler Injections. The Aesthetic Guide. September/October 2012, Volume 15, Number 5, p. 58

20. Garcia R. and Garcia A. The Use of Microcannulas in Facial Volume Restoration Treatment with Poly-L-Lactic Acid. Surg Cosmet Dermatol. 2011; 3(1)74-6

21. Cohen J., Berlin A. Integrating Cannulas into Your Filler Practice. The Dermatologist 2012; 20(6): (/issue/2367)

22. Brody, H. J. Use of Hyaluronidase in the Treatment of Granulomatous Hyaluronic Acid Reactions or Unwanted Hyaluronic Acid Misplacement. Dermatol Surg. 2008 Jan;34(1):135. https://www.ncbi.nlm.nih.gov/pubmed/16042932

23. 2018 Plastic Surgery Statistics Report, American Society for Aesthetic Plastic Surgery (ASAPS). Available at https://www.surgery.org/sites/default/files/ASAPS-Stats2018_0.pdf pg 11 [Last assessed 7/3/19]

24. Steven H. Dayan, MD, Benjamin A. Bassichis, MD. Facial Dermal Fillers: Selection of Appropriate Products and Techniques. Aesthetic Surgery Journal, Volume 28, Issue 3, May 2008, Pages 335–347, https://doi.org/10.1016/j.asj.2008.03.004

25. Bohluli, Behnam; Aghagoli, Mehran; Sarkarat, Farzin; Malekzadeh, Mansour; and Moharamnejad, Nima. Facial Sculpturing by Fat Grafting. Available at: http://cdn. intechopen.com/pdfs-wm/44956.pdf (Last Assessed 24 March 2016)

26. Cohen, Joel L. et al. Treatment of Hyaluronic Acid Filler-Induced Impending Necrosis with Hyaluronidase: Consensus Recommendations

27. Lamb, Jerome Paul, and Christopher Chase Surek. Facial Volumization an Anatomic Approach, p. 3, 20. Thieme, 2018

28. Kim, Hee-Jin, et al. Clinical Anatomy of the Face for Filler and Botulinum Toxin Injection. 2016 pg 21, 49

29. AccuVein. Available at https://www.accuvein.com/why-accuvein/evidence/ [Last assessed 21 June 2019]

30. Hibiclens. 3455 Hibiclens US Patient Booklet 8pp_9.23.16.pdf. Available at http://monlyckeus.wpengine.com/wp-content/uploads/2019/03/Guide-to-Inpatient-Bathing-with-Hibiclens.pdf [Last assessed 21 June 2019]

31. Lasercyn. Available at https://otc.intraderm.com/products/lasercyn-dermal-spray-8-oz.html [Last assessed 21 June 2019]

32. Rong, A., et al,. 0.01 % Hypochlorous Acid as an Alternative Skin Antiseptic: An In Vitro Comparison. ©2018 by the American Society for Dermatologic Surgery.Pub. Wolters Kluwer. 2018. p. 1489-1493.

33. Lee, G. TSK STERiGLIDE Microcannula Techniques Video. Available at https://www.air-titeaesthetics.com/tsk-steriglide. ©2013 [Assessed 6/29/19]

34. Clague, M, and Goodman, G. A Rethink on Hyaluronidase Injection, Intra-arterial Injection, and Blindness: Is There Another Option for Treatment of Retinal Artery Embolism Caused by Intra-arterial Injection of Hyaluronic Acid. Derm Surg 2016 Apr; 42(4):547-9

35. Carey W. Weinkle S. Retraction of the Plunger on a Syringe of Hyaluronic Acid Before Injection: Are We Safe? ©2015 by the American Society for Dermatologic Surgery. Inc. Published by Wolters Kluwer Health, Inc. p. S340-S346

36. Torbeck R, Schwarcz R., et al. In Vitro Evaluation of Preinjection Aspiration for Hyaluronic Fillers as Safety Checkpoint. © 2019 by the American Society for Dermatologic Surgery Inc. p. 1-5

37. Casabona, Gabriela. Blood Aspiration Test for Cosmetic Fillers to Prevent Accidental Intravascular Injection in the Face. Dermatologic Surgery: July 2018 -Vol. 41, Issue 7, pg 841-847

38. Van Loghem, J., Fouche, J., and Thuis, J. Sensitivity of Aspiration as a Safety Test Before Injections of Soft Tissue Fillers. Journal of Cosmetic Dermatology; Vol 17; Issuie 1; Feb 2018, pg. 39-46

39. Lee, G. Mid-Face Volume Replacement. MedEsthetics. March 2014, Volume 10, Number 2, p. 22-26

40. Lee, Garry. Lovely Lips: MedEsthetics. Jan/Feb 2017, Vol 13, Number 1, pg. 54

41. Lee, Garry. PRiME Internatonal Journal of Aesthetic and Anti-Ageing Medicine. Jan/Feb 2015; Vol 5, Issue 1;, pg. 29

42. Sadick NS1, Bosniak SL, Cantisano-Zilkha M, Glavas IP, Roy D. Definition of the Tear Trough and the Tear Trough rating scale. J Cosmet Dermatol. 2007 Dec; 6 (4):218-22

43. Funt D., Pavivic T. Dermal Fillers in Aesthetics: an Overview of Adverse Events and Treatment Approaches. Clinical, Cosmetic and Investigational

Dermatology 2013; 6: 303-310

44. Thanasarnaksorn, W. et al. Severe Vision Loss Caused by Cosmetic Filler Augmentation: Case Series with Review of Cause and Therapy. J Cosmet Dermatol. 2018; 1-7

45. Sharad J. Dermal Fillers for the Treatment of Tear Trough Deformity: A Review of Anatomy, Treatment Techniques, and Their Outcomes. Journal of Cutaneous and Aesthetic Surgery. 2012; 5(4): 229-238

46. Smit R. Rejuvenating the Periorbital Area: Lower Eyelid, Tear Trough, and Mid-Face. Injectable Treatments. 2013. Available at: https:// www. prime-journal.com/rejuvenating-the-periorbital-area-lower-eyelid-%E2%80%A8tear-trough-and-mid-face-%E2%80%A8/ [Last assessed 19 September 2014]

47. Hylenex. https://hylenex.com/advancing-the-science/ [Last assessed 19 June 2019]

48. Carruthers, Jean, et al. Soft Tissue Augmentation. 4th ed., Elsevier, 2018; pg 115-121, 185-188

49. McCrudden, MT; McAlister, E.; Courtenay, AJ.; Gonzalez-Vazquez, P.; Singh, TR.; Donelly, RF. Microneedle applications in improving skin appearance

50. Lee, Garry R. Opening Channels. MedEsthetics Jan/Feb 2017 pg 32

51. Smith, PA. Intra-articular Autologous Conditioned Plasma Injections Provide Safe and Efficacious Treatment for Knee Osteoarthritis: An FDA-Sanctioned, Randomized, Double-blind, Placebo-controlled Clinical Trial

52. Comert, Killic S.; Gungormus, M.; Sumbullu, MA. Is Arthrocentesis Plus Platelet-Rich Plasma Superior to Arthrocentesis Alone in the Treatment of Temporomandibular Joint Osteoarthritis? A Randomized Clinical Trial

53. Lee, G. and Sasaki, G. PRP for Hair Loss. MedEsthetics. September 2014, Volume 10, Number 6, p. 28-32

54. Journal of Cosmetic and Laser Therapy. Treatment of Striae Distensae Combined Enhanced Penetration Platelet-Rich Plasma and Ultrasound after Plasma Fractional Radiofrequency. Pub. 21 March 2016. Dong-Hye Suh , Sang-Jun Lee , Jong-Ho Lee , Hyun-Ju Kim, Min-Kyung Shin , Kye-Yong Song. 10.3109/14764172.2012.738916T.

55. Skinfinity RF. Available at: https://www.deviceinformed.com/medical-devices-global-directory/secondary-care/dermatology-aesthetic-medicine/radiofrequency-generators/skinfinity-rf [Last assessed 2 July 2019]

56. Kim, C., Park, S. Seo, J. Chang. Clinical Experience with Hyaluronic Acid Filler Complications. Journal of Plastic Reconstructive &Aesthetic Surgery (2011) 64, 892-897

57. Silverstein, S. et al. Hyaluronidase in Opthalmology. Journal of Applied Research, Vol 12, No. 1, 2012

58. Carruthers, Jean, et al. Soft Tissue Augmentation. 4th ed., Elsevier, 2018; pg 97-99

59. D. Kim, E. Yoon, et al. Vascular Complications of Hyaluronic Acid Fillers and the Role of Hyaluronidase in Management. Journal of Plastic, Reconstructive, & Aesthetic Surgery (2011) 64, 169-173, 1590-1595

60. Toscano F. Reversal of Skin Necrosis Caused by Facial Artery Occlusion. http://regenerativemedicinenow.com, ©2017

61. DeLorenzi C. New High Dose Pulsed Hyaluronidase Protocol for Hyaluronic Acid Filler Vascular Adverse Events. Aesthetic Surgery Journal 2017, ©2017 Vol 37 p. 814-825

62. Zhu, G., et al,. Efficacy of Retrobulbar Hyaluronidase Injection for Vision Loss Resulting from Hyaluronic Acid Filler Embolization. Aesthetic Surgery Journal. ©2018, Vol 38. P. 12-22

63. Chestnut, Cameron. Restoration of Visual Loss with Retrobulbar Hyaluronidase Injection After Hyaluronic Acid Filler. Dermatologic Surgery; 2017;0:1-3

64. Carruthers, Jean, et al. Soft Tissue Augmentation. 4th ed., Elsevier, 2018; pg 200, 215-226, 236-237

65. Cohen, MD. Understanding, Avoiding, and Managing Dermal Filler Complications. Dermatol Surg 2008;34:592-599

66. Pro-Nox. http://www.carestreamamerica.com/pro-nox/ [Last assessed 19 June 2018]

67. Brotzman E. Sandoval L,. et al. Use of Nitrous Oxide in Dermatology: A Systematic Review. © 2018 by the American Society for Dermatologic Surgery, Inc. Published by Wolters Kluwer Health, Inc. p. 661-669

68. Carrie Strom – Allergan Senior VP US Medical Aesthetics, lecture at The Aesthetic Forum, 2 March 2019

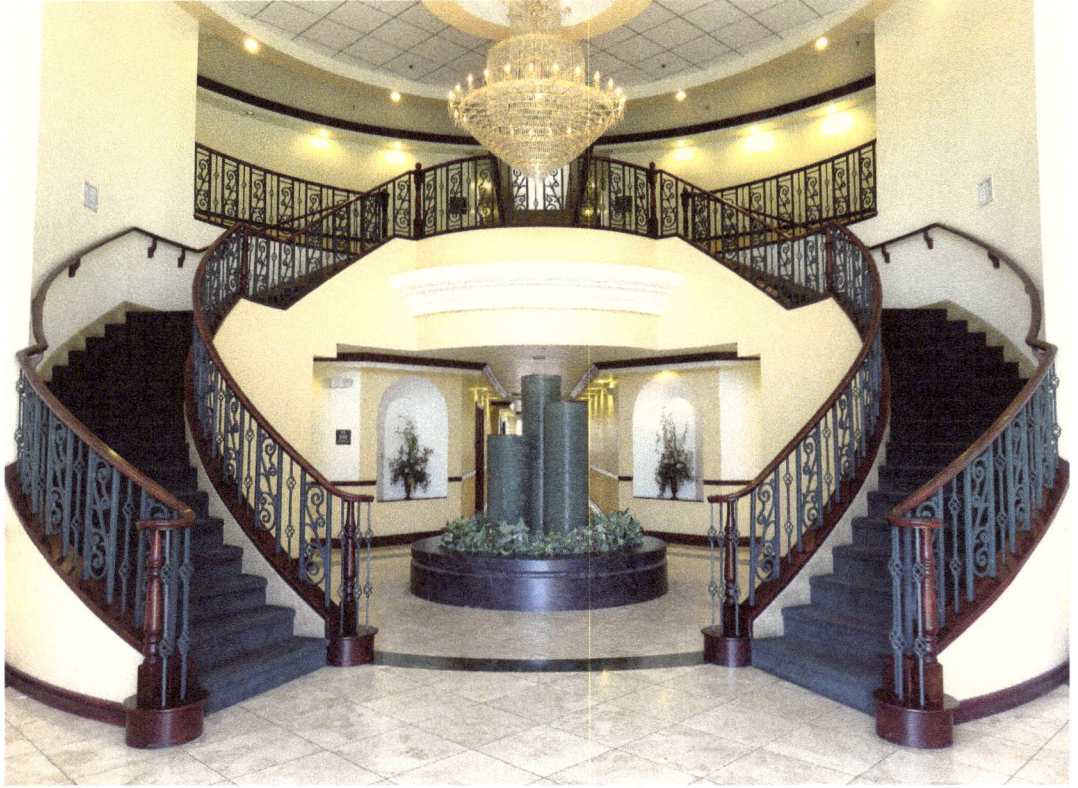

* 9 7 8 0 5 7 8 5 2 8 7 4 8 *